Dedication

To my many dear patients, who have become my friends.
They have honoured me with their cooperation, faith and
acceptance of my efforts and my limitations.

Since writing this book a personal experience has given
me an even closer understanding of some of the difficulties
and anxieties that they have had to face.

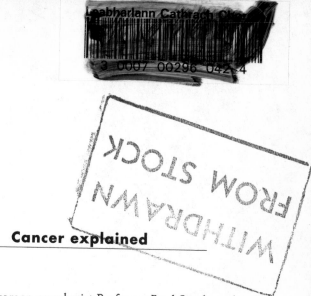

Cancer explained

Throughout his career, oncologist Professor Fred Stephens has won numerous honours and awards. He was a Fulbright fellow and has been visiting Professor at many overseas universities and cancer hospitals as well as a number in Australia. He has been dedicated to medical education and research with a special interest in prevention and early detection and treatment of cancers as well as combined and integrated treatment of advanced cancers. In recent years he has been President of the International Society for Regional Cancer Therapy. A prolific author, his articles and chapters on cancer have been published in many Australian and overseas journals and books.

Cancer explained

Frederick O. Stephens

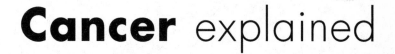

AM MD MS FRCS(Ed) FACS FRACS

Professor of Surgical Oncology

and Former Head of Department of Surgery

The University of Sydney

and Consultant Surgeon Emeritus of Surgical Oncology

The Royal Prince Alfred Hospital, Sydney

Newleaf

Newleaf
an imprint of
Gill & Macmillan Ltd
Goldenbridge
Dublin 8
with associated companies throughout the world
© Frederick Stephens, 1997

This edition is published by arrangement with Wakefield Press, Australia.

0 7171 2793 1

Printed by ColourBooks Ltd, Dublin

A catalogue record is available for this book from the British Library.

1 3 5 4 2

Contents

PART ONE
Questions commonly asked about cancer

PART TWO
Tests and treatments for cancer

PART THREE
Some common cancers

PART FOUR
Where do we go from here?

Foreword
by Dr James Wright

At long last, we have a comprehensive, readable and understandable book on cancer. A book that does not scare, but puts the entire topic in its true perspective. *Cancer Explained* helps remove much of the mystique, horror and hopelessness that many people associate with cancer. This book is filled with page after page of good cheer, as we see countless ways in which everyone can take steps – usually simple ones – to help prevent the disease from striking. That is marvellous news in itself. Although most of these steps have been known for years, they are brought together in *Cancer Explained* in an easily followed way. Then we are gently walked through the various forms of cancer, the signs and symptoms which should alert us, the steps the doctor will take in diagnosis and treatment. Finally there are simple explanations of the litany of cancer-related words.

Cancer Explained is filled with common sense, empathy, and hard-hitting facts, all wrapped up in words that anyone can follow and understand. Western medicine still offers the most important option in dealing with cancer. But the book shows an appreciation of the enormous range of 'alternative' methods of prevention and treatment. Many accepted forms of western medicine are based on naturally occurring products. Fred Stephens acknowledges the proliferating data on fibre, isoflavinoids, phyto-estrogens, and their value in prevention – a reason why cancer is so rare in countries where legumes and other high-fibre, low-fat foods are part of the everyday diet. There are lessons to be learned from all parts of the globe.

Fred Stephens has a long and distinguished association with cancer and education, at the University of Sydney, Sydney Hospital and The Royal Prince Alfred Hospital. For many years he educated, advised and treated vast numbers of students and patients. All have benefited from his experience and, just as importantly, his understanding and empathy for his fellow human beings.

I am intrigued by this fine book, and recommend it to medical people as well as everyone out there. Reading this book will help you better understand all aspects of the second-largest killer in our community. And it will help you save lives, most importantly your own, or that of family or friends.

Read this book, and tell your friends to read it also. I am certainly recommending it to my media audience.

Dr James Wright

Preface

My intention in writing this book has been to answer the questions that patients and friends ask me about cancer. It is intended to help not only cancer patients or friends or family of cancer patients, but also nurses and paramedical personnel. The book should also help medical practitioners to answer patients' questions and perhaps give them a broader understanding of the various aspects of cancer.

Section 1 will be of interest to all people concerned about cancer. It describes what cancer means, what is known about its causes, who is at risk and how it might be prevented.

Section 2 describes the general and local features of cancer, test procedures, special investigations that might be helpful and what the patient might expect in having these investigations carried out. It also outlines the different forms of treatment that are available.

Section 3 deals with specific types of cancer in different parts of the body. Readers may wish to read only that part which is of particular concern to them.

Section 4 is a short review of possible new challenges and likely advances in cancer treatment in the future.

A glossary and an index provide a cross-reference to all sections.

I hope that this book will not only give the lay reader a better understanding of the problems of cancer, but also help all who care for people with cancer. It is only by promoting a better understanding of the clinical realities and the therapeutic possibilities of cancer that the social and emotional needs of patients and those who love and care for them will be met.

Author's note

I wish to acknowledge the inspiration given to me by the dedicated work of many colleagues and friends, both in the medical and in the nursing professions but also in the research, secretarial and administrative fields, both in Australia and overseas. Many have been in the forefront of present-day success stories in the care of people with cancer but have often been taken for granted. Such successes include the change in management of patients with melanoma: in my student days this was a disease with an 80% mortality rate; the reduction of the mortality rate to less than 20% in present-day Australian clinics has been part of the everyday life and work of my close friends and colleagues at the Sydney Melanoma Unit.

To see the much improved results of treatment of locally advanced sarcomas in limbs without the need for limb amputation in eight out of ten patients who would previously have been subject to amputation has been a true source of inspiration.

This improvement has also been largely due to the cooperation and dedicated work of close colleagues.

To see governments and other authorities at long last acknowledge the risk of tobacco smoking and introduce measures to reduce the general exposure of non-smokers to tobacco smoke and more especially to discourage young people from taking up the habit, has been the result of constant prompting by dedicated colleagues.

These are just some examples of the quality of work of many good people which is often hardly recognised or acknowledged.

Finally, I am proud to acknowledge the help and understanding of my family and friends. My family has always given encouragement and support in my work, even though it has often meant the absence of their husband, father, grandfather, brother, uncle or cousin from other activities. My friends have also been understanding and helpful. Both groups helped in the writing of this book by insisting that it be written in terms they readily understood.

Questions commonly asked about cancer

What is cancer?

The word 'cancer' is a Latin word meaning 'crab'. The condition was called cancer in ancient times because an advanced cancer was thought to resemble a crab with claws reaching out into surrounding tissues. A cancer, or malignant growth, is now known to be a continuous, purposeless, unwanted and uncontrolled growth of cells.

Although most normal body tissues contain cells that have the ability to grow or reproduce, they do so only when there is a need: when the need has been satisfied, the growth stops. For example, cells in some tissues such as the skin or blood wear out quickly and are constantly being replaced. Cells reproduce only to meet the immediate needs of the body. However, in the case of a cancer, cell reproduction continues for no good reason, and excessive numbers of abnormal cells are produced – there is no 'switching off' mechanism. The abnormal and unwanted cells spread into surrounding tissues, causing damage. The abnormal cancer cells also tend to invade blood and lymph vessels, where they may travel to other parts of the body and establish new colonies of growing cells. These colonies are called secondary (or 'metastatic') cancers.

A cancer is quite different from an infection. An infection is caused when germs or organisms from outside the body invade body tissues, causing damage. The body's defences recognise the germs as foreign material and establish protective measures to destroy these invading organisms. Invading cancer cells, on the other hand, are abnormal cells that have developed from the body's own cells. They are thus not recognised by the body's defences as being foreign, and tend to grow and invade without being attacked by this defence mechanism.

A growth of cells that seems to be under some sort of control is called a benign tumour. Although there is no apparent purpose in the growth, the cells are more mature and closely resemble the cells of the tissue from which they developed. Once the growth reaches a certain size, it usually slows down or stops growing any further. All the cells of a benign tumour stay together as a lump or swelling that is usually confined by a capsule or lining of fibrous tissue. They do not spread to other parts of the body.

With cancer or malignant growth, on the other hand, the cells look abnormal and less like the cells from which they developed. As a rule, the more malignant the tumour the more abnormal the cells appear. The multiplication of cells also continues without control, causing the tumour to get bigger and bigger. The tumour invades surrounding body tissues, increasing the likelihood of it spreading to other parts of the body and establishing secondary growths.

TYPES OF CANCER

Although all malignant growths are commonly referred to as cancers, the word cancer (or 'carcinoma') is more correctly applied to a malignant growth of glandular cells or cells lining a hollow organ or a duct, or cells lining skin surfaces. For example, a cancer may start in cells lining the mouth, throat, stomach or bowel, cells lining the ducts of the breast, cells lining the air passages in the lungs or cells lining the cavity of the uterus or vagina, the kidney or bladder. Glandular cancers may develop in the thyroid gland, the prostate gland, the glandular tissue of the breast, the pancreas or the salivary glands. Similar cancers may also develop in cells of certain organs such as the liver or the kidneys.

Malignant tumours of these glands or of lining cells are truly called cancers and are the most common forms of malignant tumour. However, sometimes cells of other tissues (such as blood, bone, the brain, or muscle) will become malignant (i.e. grow continuously, without purpose and without control or restraint). Although these are commonly called cancers, they are more correctly called by other names, as described in Section 3 of this book.

Are all tumours malignant?

The answer is 'no'. Non-malignant or benign tumours are, in general, much more common than malignant tumours.

Is cancer always dangerous?

If a cancer is detected early, while it is still small and before it has spread to another part of the body, it can usually be completely removed surgically, or destroyed in some other way so that it is eradicated or cured before any serious damage has been done.

Cancers are dangerous when they cause damage and destruction to surrounding tissues and when they spread to other organs and tissues where they establish secondary cancers. The secondary growths damage and interfere with the function of the organ or tissue in which they are growing. For example, secondary cancers in the liver interfere with the function of the liver; secondary cancers in the lung block the air passages and interfere with breathing, causing lung infection or pneumonia; secondary cancers in the brain will cause pressure on the brain and interfere with its function; and those in bones often cause pain and weakness of the bones, which may then collapse or break.

How common is cancer?

Cancer is known to occur in all societies and in all parts of the world. It affects animals as well as humans. Cancer is known to have been present in ancient as well as in modern times. However, the types of cancer most prevalent in a community vary with the age, sex and race of those in the community, as well as their geographical location, the economic and environmental situation and their diet and lifestyle.

Although in westernised societies cancer is responsible for about 25% of deaths, it is less commonly a cause of death than heart and vascular disease, which is the greatest cause of death, especially among older people. Young people in our society are much more at risk from accidents at home or on the road. Cancer is relatively uncommon among young people.

What causes cancer?

For generations doctors, researchers, philosophers and quacks have been trying to find a single cause for all cancers, and consequently a single cure. No such cause has been found and probably none exists as such. There are many different factors that start changes in cells which lead to cancer. It is not known whether these factors all eventually act through a final common pathway in changing a biochemical 'triggering' action in the cell. One possibility is that rather than stimulating changes in cells causing them to reproduce indiscriminately, the cancer factors weaken the body defences against cells that have a natural tendency to reproduce continuously. (That is, rather than stimulating cells by applying an accelerator mechanism, the possibility is that they interfere with the body's natural ability to apply a 'braking' mechanism to cell growth.) Most recent studies suggest a combination of these theories may be correct. Cells contain genes (controlling chemical particles) that 'switch on' a self-limiting repair process when a tissue is injured. After repair the healing mechanism is switched off. Cancer-causing agents such as certain viruses (retrovirus) may change some genes so that they continue to cause cell reproduction. These are called oncogenes. The oncogenes change the nature of the life-giving protein component of the cell (DNA or deoxyribonucleic acid) so that the switch-on mechanism or repair continues and is not switched off. There is evidence that some people have abnormal oncogenes in their cell genetic make-up and that these abnormal oncogenes predispose those affected to a greater risk of developing cancer.

Many different factors are known to result in different types of cancers. In our society, **tobacco smoking** is responsible for an increased incidence of cancers of the lung, mouth, throat and larynx as well as cancers of the oesophagus, stomach, pancreas, kidney, bladder and even the breast.

ve ultra-violet light from **sunshine** is responsible for a
...creased incidence of skin cancers, especially in fair-
skinned people who live in sunny tropical or sub-tropical
climates.

Some **industrial irritants and chemical carcinogens**
(cancer-causing substances) cause different types of cancers. The
first cancer found in Western countries to be caused by a
chemical agent was cancer of the scrotum, which commonly
developed in chimney sweeps in Britain in the eighteenth
century. The cause was found to be soot which collected in the
scrotal area in those industrial workers. Later, certain dyes used
by German workers in chemical factories and excreted in the
urine were found to be associated with an increased incidence of
bladder cancer. People using phosphorus to paint luminous dials
on clocks and watches were also found to have a high incidence
of bone cancer. The phosphorus was absorbed through the
workers' habit of wetting the tips of their small phosphorous
paintbrushes by dipping them in their mouths. A number of
chemical agents cause cancer in experimental animals. Similar
agents are present in tobacco tars and products of the petro-
leum industry and other chemical industries.

Viruses have often been studied as a possible cause for
human cancer. This belief has been based on evidence that
certain viruses cause cancers in animals and that in humans,
warts are known to be caused by a virus. (A wart is a benign
tumour.) However, apart from a few exceptions, there is no clear
evidence that viruses are responsible for cancer in humans. The
exceptions include a certain cancer in the back of the nose, most
common in Chinese who live in or near the Kwangtung province
of China near Hong Kong. In these people there is a high incidence of infection with the Epstein-Barr virus, which may play a
part in developing this cancer. The malignant tumour Burkitt's

lymphoma, most common in certain parts of Africa, is also associated with a high incidence of infection with the same or a similar virus.

It is also a common observation that **pre-existing abnormalities in tissue** are more likely to develop malignant cells than normal tissues. Abnormal tissues include congenitally abnormal tissues, chronically irritated tissues, chronically wasted or worn out (atrophic) tissues, chronically inflamed or severely scarred tissues or tissues with one or more surface sores (ulcers). Pre-existing benign tumours such as lumps under the surface lining of skin or mouth or lumps projecting from such a surface (polyps or papillomas) have an increased chance of malignant change.

The habits of **chewing betel nut or tobacco leaf** are responsible for a highly increased incidence of cancer in the mouth of people who live in countries such as India or New Guinea where these habits are common.

Who is at risk?

Although the risk of developing cancer is much less in young people than in older people, cancer can affect people of any age, race or occupation in any part of the world. People who have been cured of one cancer often ask about the risk of developing a second cancer. People who have been cured of one type of cancer have a slightly increased risk of developing a cancer not only of the same system but of another system of the body in comparison to people who have never been affected, but the increased risk is quite small. Most never develop a second cancer unless they continue to indulge in an obvious cancer-causing habit such as cigarette smoking.

Is cancer contagious?

No, there is no evidence that, in the normal course of events, cancer can be passed from one individual to another. Liver cancer is not infectious but a common cause of liver cancer is hepatitis B or hepatitis C. These hepatitis infections do spread easily from person to person, mainly from food or intimate contact, so that liver cancer develops more commonly in people who have been infected.

AIDS (acquired immune deficiency syndrome) is caused by a virus infection and may predispose a person to cancer, but it is not itself a cancer. In this disease the sufferer's natural immune defences against both infection and cancer are damaged, resulting in a high incidence of infection and also a high incidence of cancer in affected people.

Does heredity play a part?

In some relatively uncommon cancers there is a strong hereditary factor; in other cancers there is a less obvious hereditary factor; but for most cancers there is no evidence of a hereditary factor at all. Among cancers with a strong hereditary factor is familial polyposis coli, a condition in which half the children of an affected parent are likely to develop the condition of multiple polyps in the large bowel. All those affected who do develop these particular polyps will eventually develop cancer in the bowel, usually by the age of 40 years.

With another rare but inherited familial condition, xeroderma pigmentosa, there is a high incidence of development of skin cancer.

More common cancers with an increased familial incidence are cancers of the breast, stomach and bowel. Although the risk is small in most families, occasionally there may be a considerably increased risk. For example, there have been rare reports of families in which about half the female blood relatives have developed breast cancer. It is not known what is responsible for this apparent increased risk in a few families. It may be strictly an inherited oncogene that affects the cells, tissues, or body defences, or it may be that members of these families are more likely to have similar habits or be affected by similar living conditions.

There is a slightly increased risk of cancer of the stomach, colon or rectum in relatives of sufferers from these conditions, but this risk is low except in those with an obvious predisposing cause such as familial polyposis coli.

Another indication of the genetic influence with stomach cancer is the fact that there have been reports of a slightly higher risk for people with blood group A than there is for people of other blood groups. Such information is well documented, but the risk is so small that it is of little practical value to anyone other than statisticians and scientists studying cancer. Many thousands of people of different blood groups would have to be studied before any difference in cancer incidence could be detected, and some studies have not detected any difference. For the individual with blood group A the risk of being any more likely to develop stomach cancer is almost negligible.

Does age play a part?

In general, the risk of developing most cancers increases with age. However, there are exceptions. Although cancer in young people is uncommon, no age group is entirely free from risk.

A certain cancer of the kidney known as a Wilm's tumour (nephroblastoma) is quite uncommon, but when it does occur it is almost always in infants less than five years of age and may even be present at birth. Other malignant tumours which, although uncommon, are more likely to occur in infants are a cancer of nerve tissue (neuroblastoma) and a type of brain cancer (medulloblastoma).

Acute leukaemias (cancers of blood cells), especially acute lymphatic leukaemia (a cancer of a special type of white blood cell), are more likely to occur in children and adolescents than in adults. Teenagers and young adults have the highest incidence of bone cancers (osteosarcomas) as well as the highest incidence of the most common type of lymphoma (cancer of the lymph glands) known as Hodgkin's disease. Burkitt's lymphoma is a tumour that predominantly affects the jaw of children, most commonly in tropical Africa and New Guinea. Bone cancers are uncommon, but when they do occur it is most often during the growth periods of children and young adults.

Malignant tumours of the testis are uncommon, but when they occur it is most often in men between the ages of 20 and 40. Ovarian cancer and cancer of the cervix of the uterus most commonly affect women between the ages of 40 and 60 years, but cancer of the body of the uterus is more likely to occur in women over 60 years of age.

Lung cancer is becoming increasingly common in communities where cigarette smoking is prevalent. It most frequently occurs between the ages of 40 and 60 years, probably because it takes some years for the irritating effects of tobacco tars to cause changes in the air passages that lead to cancer.

Breast cancer may affect women of any age but is uncommon in women under 30 years. Thereafter it increases in incidence with increasing age, having a mean incidence of about 60 years.

The incidence of stomach and bowel cancers increases with age, reaching a peak between 60 and 75 years of age.

Cancer of the prostate gland is also a disease of increasing age. It is not often seen in men under 50, but is the most common internal cancer affecting men over 65 years.

Skin cancers (except melanoma) and mouth and throat cancers become more common with increasing age, although the sun damage to skin may have occurred many years before. Melanoma, on the other hand, occurs in people of all age groups, although it is rare before puberty. Unlike other skin cancers, which most often occur on the face because that skin is most constantly exposed to the sun, melanoma is not so directly related to prolonged sunlight exposure. Melanoma occurs most commonly on the parts of the body and lower limbs that are not constantly exposed to the sun but are more likely to have been damaged by occasional episodes of sunburn.

Are some people more likely to develop cancer than others?

Clearly, the answer to this is 'yes'. Although a lot of cancers develop 'out of the blue', so to speak, in tissues that were apparently otherwise normal, many cancers develop in tissues that were not previously normal. Abnormal tissues are more likely to develop malignant change.

Repeated **sun damage** to skin is often followed by thickening and crustiness of the surface layers of the skin called 'hyperkeratosis'. This is a pre-malignant condition and usually precedes the development of skin cancer. Hyperkeratosis of the lips also predisposes to cancer on the lips, especially the lower lip. Melanoma commonly develops in a pre-existing mole, or pigmented naevus.

People who have **pernicious anaemia** (a blood disorder) or **chronic atrophic gastritis** (a stomach disorder) have a six times greater risk of developing stomach cancer than other people. Stomach ulcers too may occasionally develop into stomach cancers, although the more common duodenal ulcer has not shown any tendency to develop into cancer.

Polyps in the large bowel (colon or rectum) predispose to an increased incidence of development of cancer in the large bowel. A chronically inflamed bowel, as in ulcerative colitis, has an increased risk of developing cancer. The younger the patient at the onset of ulcerative colitis, the longer it has been present, and the greater the extent of the colitis in the colon, the greater the risk of cancer developing. The risk of cancer developing in another chronic inflammatory condition of the bowel, granular colitis (Crohn's disease), is also increased, but not to the same degree as in ulcerative colitis.

Chronic irritation of the lining of the mouth and throat, as seen especially in smokers and sometimes in diabetics, may lead to a thickening of the surface cell layer that shows as white patches (leukoplakia). These white patches also have a definite predisposition towards the development of cancer.

Cancer of the gall bladder is not common, but when it does occur it is almost always in a gall bladder containing stones with chronic irritation and inflammation in the wall of the gall bladder. The same applies to cancers of the kidney and the bladder, which are more common in people with longstanding kidney or bladder stones than in others.

Any **chronic inflammation** of tissue can predispose to cancer.

In fact, any chronically inflamed, chronically irritated or injured, or chronically degenerate (atrophic) tissue has a some-what increased risk of developing cancer after some years. These include chronically discharging wounds, burn scars, or varicose ulcers in the lower legs, which only rarely develop malignant change, as well as the chronically irritated lining of the mouth, throat, and air passages of smokers in which malignant change is relatively common. Although it is true that women who have chronic mastitis in the breasts (more correctly known as benign mammary dysplasia, hormonal mastopathy or fibroadenosis cystica) do have a slightly higher risk of developing breast cancer, the increased risk is very small.

Whether malignancy follows **acute injury** is somewhat less clear. However, there are incidences where tumours, especially sarcomas (cancers in bone or muscle), have been found in tissues after some well-documented injury such as a kick in the thigh or calf, or a blow to a bone at football. Whether the tumour followed the injury or whether the injury simply drew attention to a tumour that was already present is often impossible to determine in any particular instance. Certainly, it is very rare indeed for a malignant tumour to follow such an injury, as these types of injury are very common and sarcomas of this type are very uncommon.

In the case of **benign tumours**, there is some risk that the tumour may become malignant. With some types of benign tumours such as warts, the risk is extremely small, virtually negligible. With the common fatty tumour called a lipoma, the risk is so small that removal of the lipoma is usually not justified. However, with others such as papilloma (a fern-like projecting tumour) in the mouth or in a duct of a breast, some soft tissue tumours, adenomas (gland lumps), or benign tumours of bone or cartilage, there is a small but somewhat greater risk of malignant change, and for many of them surgical removal of the lump is usually recommended. With still other benign tumours, such as polyps of the stomach or colon or especially papilloma of the rectum, the risk of malignant change is of real significance and surgical removal of these tumours is virtually always indicated.

Congenitally abnormal tissue also has a greater risk of malignant change than normal tissue. For example, a thyroglossal cyst (a congenital remnant of thyroid tissue high in the neck or in the back of the tongue), a branchial cyst (a cyst resulting from a congenital developmental abnormality in the neck) or an undescended testis (in which the testis had not descended into the scrotum at birth) will have an increased risk of developing cancer than normally developed tissues. These increased risks are of varying degrees. The risk is very small in the case of branchial cysts, but quite high in the case of an undescended testis.

Does gender play a part?

Obviously, cancers that occur in organs of one sex only are unique to that sex. However, breast cancer, although 100 times more common in women, occasionally develops in the male breast. When it does occur in males it tends to be more aggressive.

The incidence of lung cancer has increased some 10 or 15 times over the past 40 years. This increase has been predominantly in men as a result of increased use of tobacco products by males. Twenty years ago, lung cancer was 10 times more common in men than in women. However, following the trend in recent years for increased use of cigarettes by women, the incidence of lung cancer of females is now approaching that of men.

Skin cancers are more prevalent in men than in women because of the increased exposure to the sun of men working and playing out of doors, often without a hat or shirt. On the other hand, many cancers have a significantly different incidence in the sexes for no apparent reason. Cancer of the stomach, for example, is three times more likely to occur in men than in women and cancer of the rectum is somewhat more common in males. On the other hand, cancer of the colon is found slightly more often in females. Cancer of the oesophagus is more common in men, especially cancer of the middle and lower oesophagus; however, cancer of the upper oesophagus is somewhat more likely to occur in women. Primary liver cancer is four times more common in men than women. For some unknown reason, the incidence of cancer of the pancreas is increasing in the USA, especially in men who smoke cigarettes. It is also being seen more frequently in women, especially those with diabetes mellitus.

Does diet play a part?

There is an association between diet and some cancers of the digestive tract. Certainly a high-fibre diet appears to be protective against bowel cancer. Whether this is a mechanical effect of the bulk of high fibre alone or some other factor is uncertain. Recent studies have shown that fibre is basically composed of a complex carbohydrate, glucan, which has been shown to have properties of stimulation of the immune (protective) system. The different incidences of cancer of some tissues (e.g. breast and prostate) between Orientals and Caucasians may also be related to diet. Traditionally Orientals have a diet with a high content of legumes (peas, soy beans etc.). Legumes have a high content of naturally occurring hormones – the phytoestrogens. Some studies suggest that this may be a factor in the relatively low incidence of breast diseases (including cancer) in Oriental females and the relatively low incidence of prostate cancer in Oriental males. This belief is supported by evidence that men and women of Asian races who are born and raised in Western countries, and Asian men and women who adopt Western diets, either in their own country or in a Western country, have a significantly increased risk of developing prostate cancer or breast cancer. This risk approaches that of Caucasians. However, for most cancers there is little real evidence that diet plays a part. There are so many variable factors among people of different population groups that it is always difficult to prove which particular factors were responsible for any difference in the incidence of cancer. For example, as well as differences in diet there may be genetic differences, racial differences, environmental differences, or differences in social habits or customs such as smoking, differences in the incidence of parasites or infections or even in occupational stress or psychological factors. However, the evidence of association between diet and cancer is strongest for cancer of the large bowel. Cancer of the oesophagus, stomach, pancreas and liver are all more common in heavy drinkers of alcohol, especially if they are smokers.

Forty or 50 years ago, cancer of the stomach was much more common in Western societies than it is today. The decreasing incidence in recent years may be associated with the increased use of refrigeration and decreased use of artificial chemical preservatives in food. It is more common in Japan than in Britain or the USA. This may be genetic or due to the high consumption of smoked fish in Japan or both. There is a higher incidence of stomach cancer in people who have a diet high in refined starch and animal fat as opposed to a lower incidence in people who have diets rich in fruit and vegetables.

Similarly, the incidence of cancer of the colon and rectum has been found to be higher in people who eat a great deal of meat and other animal fats and refined foods compared to people who eat little animal fat or refined food but have a high intake of crude fibre and roughage. More recently, a high consumption of animal fat has also been found to be associated with an increased incidence of breast cancer.

There have been theories that various vitamins may be protective against cancer. Although some of the claims of protection and cure with vitamins are probably exaggerated, there is some evidence that vitamins A and C may offer some protection.

Members of the Seventh Day Adventist church have a lower-than-average incidence of most cancers, including cancers of the lung, oesophagus, stomach, pancreas, colon and rectum. However, as well as being vegetarians with a high fibre and low meat and animal fat consumption, these people are usually non-smokers and non-consumers of alcohol, which may well be more significant. A study of male members of the Seventh Day Adventist church is of interest. It was found that those church members whose diet included meat, eggs, cheese and milk had a greater incidence of cancer of the prostate than those who abstained from all animal products.

Does race play a part?

Certainly, some cancers are more prevalent in people of some races than others. Whether the significant factor is a genetic or racial factor or whether it is more likely to be due to environmental factors, habits, or other influences such as the general health and age of the people, is hard to determine.

Some examples of increased racial incidence are the higher incidence of stomach cancer in Japan, Korea, Scandinavia, Holland and Czechoslovakia, the high incidence of cancer of the oesophagus in certain African tribes (including the Bantu in South Africa) but not the white population, the high incidence of liver cancer (hepatoma) in Malaysians and Africans, the high incidence of cancer of the post-nasal space in Chinese, especially from the Kwangtung province of China and even in their descendants born outside China, and the high incidence of both breast cancer and large bowel cancer in Europeans and people of European descent.

The high incidence of melanoma and other skin cancers in northern Europeans and especially people of northern European descent who live in tropical and sub-tropical climates is due to the genetic factor of fair skin plus the environmental factor of sunshine.

In Israel, a country with one of the highest incidences of thyroid cancer, the disease is more common among Jews born in

Europe than in those born in Asia. In South Africa, Bantus have a much higher incidence of thyroid cancer than do black Africans from other regions.

It therefore seems that, although there are genetic influences that may predispose people of different races to different cancers, it is hard to know with any particular cancer whether the most significant factors are genetic factors or habits, or diet, or result from economic or other influences.

Does geographical location play a part?

Although the incidence of a particular type of cancer varies from country to country and even within the one country according to geographical conditions, it is often difficult to be sure whether the difference is due to geographical or climatic elements, to race, to habits, to other environmental differences, or to combinations of these.

The association of skin cancer and melanoma with fair-skinned people living in a sunny climate is obvious. The incidence is highest in fair-skinned people living in sunny climates in Australia and in the sunny southern parts of the USA. Australia not only has the world's highest incidence of skin cancer and melanoma but the incidence varies from state to state according to proximity to the equator. For the more common forms of skin cancer (squamous and basal cell carcinoma) the incidence is directly related to areas of skin most exposed to the sun. Melanomas are most common on the body in men and on the thighs and lower limbs in women. Clearly, for melanoma the cause is not only the amount of direct exposure of skin to sunlight. Some other factor associated with living in a sunny climate must play a part – one of which is skin damage caused by acute sunburn, especially if episodes of sunburn occurred in childhood.

Primary cancer of the liver (hepatoma) is common in South-East Asia and East African countries but whether there is a racial predisposition or a dietary or some other environmental factor is not known, although it is known that longstanding infection with hepatitis B or C are significant causes. The cause of the high incidence of stomach cancer in Japan and Korea is uncertain but may be genetic, dietary or a combination of these factors.

Does environment play a part?

Although for most cancers there is no apparent environmental factor, there are some obvious situations where environment plays a part in causing cancer. The most obvious of these is the high incidence of skin cancers and melanoma among the white populations of Australia and the southern regions of the USA, caused by exposure to **sunshine**.

In Western societies, city dwellers living with **air pollution** have been found to have a slightly higher incidence of lung cancer than their country cousins. This factor, however, is not nearly as significant as the smoking habits of the people concerned.

The increased incidence of leukaemia in the survivors of Hiroshima and Nagasaki atom bomb explosions indicates the environmental effect of **irradiation** as a cause of this disease.

The tumour called Burkitt's lymphoma, which predominantly affects the native children in tropical Africa and New Guinea, is most common where **mosquitoes** are common and malaria is rife. There is some evidence to suggest that a mosquito carrier may play a part in spreading whatever is the cause – probably a virus.

Cancer of the thyroid is rather more common in communities where goitres are common. Goitre (or thyroid gland enlargement) is most common in places where there is a deficiency of iodine in local food and water supplies. Such places are known as '**goitre belts**' and are usually to be found in mountainous regions where iodine has been washed out of the soil over thousands or millions of years. Such areas are found in the Swiss Alps, the Rocky Mountains, the Andes, the Himalayas and the mountainous regions of New Guinea, Australia and New Zealand. The Great Lakes district in the USA is also a goitre belt. It is likely that the iodine has been washed out of the soil in the region into the Great Lakes and is lost through the rivers into the sea.

Does occupation play a part?

Present-day industrial laws protect workers against most industrial dangers including the risks of exposure to cancer-causing agents. Before the effect of environment was understood, a number of cancers were linked with working conditions but these have now been largely eliminated. For example, in the early days of X-rays, when doctors and technicians would hold the plates with bare hands, exposing them to repeated doses of radiation, there was a high incidence of skin cancer developing in the irradiated hands.

In more recent times, asbestos workers were found to have a high incidence of developing lung cancer (especially if they were also smokers) and also a highly malignant tumour of the lining of the lungs or abdominal organs called a mesothelioma. Stringent improvements to working conditions have now been introduced to protect these workers.

Another less obvious risk is the increased incidence of cancer in the air passages behind and around the nose (the para-nasal sinuses) in woodworkers, leather workers and metal workers, especially nickel workers. This is probably due to constantly breathing small particles of these materials. There is also said to be an increased risk of cancer of the larynx in people who misuse their voices, such as old time bookmakers who would shout a great deal in calling the odds, and in clergymen who spend long periods using a high-pitched chant. However, these risks would be very small compared to the risk of cigarette smokers developing the same sort of cancer.

Do habits and lifestyle play a part?

Certainly the most obvious carcinogen in present-day society is tobacco. The habit of **cigarette smoking** outweighs all other known influences as a cause of serious cancer in men and women. The incidence of lung cancer is increased some eight to 10 times in smokers compared to non-smokers, and the risk is directly related to the amount of tobacco smoked and inhaled. In the past, the rapidly increasing incidence of lung cancer was most obvious in men, but in more recent years, with increasing numbers of women smoking, the increase is now more obvious in women.

Cancers of the mouth and throat are also closely associated with the smoking habit. It is estimated that heavy smokers have about six times the risk of developing cancer in the mouth and throat than non-smokers. The risk is increased to 15 times if the smokers are also heavy drinkers.

In the case of lung cancer the risk appears to be greater in cigarette smokers than in pipe or cigar smokers, whereas with mouth cancers there is no apparent difference whether the smokers use cigarettes, pipes or cigars. Tobacco smoke is more likely to be inhaled into the lungs by cigarette smokers, but there is a similar risk of tobacco products entering the mouth with all forms of smoking.

A number of other cancers have been found to have increased incidence in smokers – these include cancer of the oesophagus, stomach, pancreas, kidney, bladder and even breast cancer.

Heavy **alcohol** drinkers, too, have an increased incidence of cancer of the mouth and throat, oesophagus, stomach, liver and pancreas. The risk is greater in those heavy drinkers who are also smokers.

Australians who spend most of their lives out of doors at work and play, on the beach and so on, are at greatest risk of developing melanoma and other skin cancers through exposure to the sun. Most young people in Australia and many other fair-skinned societies delight in developing a 'suntan'.

The habit of some Asian and Oriental people of **chewing betel nut** or tobacco leaf is associated with increased incidence of cancer of the cheek lining.

The incidence of breast cancer is lowest in women who have given birth to babies at an early age. In communities where the custom is for women to marry early and have their first babies while they are still in their teens, the incidence of breast cancer is low, while in westernised societies where first babies are commonly born to women over the age of 30 years, the incidence of breast cancer is higher. There may also be some protection against breast cancer by prolonged breastfeeding as is common in most undeveloped countries, although the evidence for this is less clear.

The association of cancer with diet and eating habits has already been mentioned (page 15).

There appears to be a direct relationship between **economic development** of a country and the incidence of large bowel cancer. In the USA it is the most common single form of cancer and in Britain it is second only to lung cancer, while in many undeveloped countries it is rarely seen. A diet high in meat, animal fats and highly refined food as in westernised, industrialised countries appears to produce cancer-inducing substances. The absence of fibre from the diet results in a relative constipation which is thought to allow these carcinogens to stay in contact with the bowel wall for prolonged periods. In undeveloped countries, in general the diet contains a great deal more roughage and fibre and less meat, fat and refined foods. This results in the passage of frequent bulky stools and a low incidence of large bowel cancer. It seems that the low carcinogen content of the stool is diluted by the bulky quantity of stool and rapidly passed by frequent bowel motions, resulting in a low incidence of large bowel cancer. There are numerous examples to support this evidence. For example, Japanese who eat the traditional high-fibre diet in Japan have a low incidence of large bowel cancer, but in Japanese who have migrated to America and changed to an American diet, the incidence of bowel cancer approaches that of Americans. Recent studies also suggest that starch-like substances called glucans may also have a protective action on the bowel wall. Glucans are found in such high-fibre foods as grains, fruit and vegetables, but there are few in fatty foods.

Naturally occurring hormones called phytoestrogens which are present in large quantities in leguminous plants such as soya beans are currently the subject of dietary studies. People who live in Asian countries where there is a high intake of these foods have a lower incidence of conditions that are common in Western societies where the intake of phytoestrogens is low. These conditions include breast diseases such as cancer, and premenstrual syndrome (PMS) as well as post menopausal symptoms in women, and prostate cancer in men.

Cultural and social customs may also have a relationship with development of cancer. Cancer of the penis is extremely rare in Jewish men, who are circumcised at birth, but is seen more frequently in Muslim men who are circumcised at about 10 years. The incidence is greatest in uncircumcised males.

Nuns have a low incidence of cancer of the cervix of the uterus but an increased incidence of breast cancer. On the other hand, cancer of the cervix is most common in prostitutes and women who commence intercourse at an early age and have had multiple male partners, as well as women who have given birth to several children.

Women who have taken the contraceptive pill for some years appear to have a somewhat reduced incidence of developing both cancer of the ovary and cancer of the uterus. On the other hand, there is evidence that prolonged use of contraceptive pills, especially the high-dose oestrogen pill, has been associated with a slightly higher risk of breast cancer. The small-dose oestrogen pill has not been shown to have any significant association with breast cancer.

Do psychological factors, stress or emotion play a part?

Among the more unusual theories about causes of cancer has been a suggestion that, as with emotional and some mental (psychosomatic) illnesses, cancer may result from an unnatural suppression of the 'fight or flight' response to anxiety or stress. It has been suggested that if a stressful situation persists over a long period and the person concerned feels that whatever action he or she takes will be wrong, a subconscious decision to escape through death by cancer may result. There is little evidence to support such a theory, although some retrospective studies have indicated that a significantly high proportion of cancer patients have experienced some form of severe stress in the period six months to two years before the onset of illness.

Most psychologists would not claim that psychological reactions are a direct cause of cancer, but some feel that they may play a part along with known chemical, genetic, environmental, viral or other causes. The association of possible psychological factors with cancer has indicated a need for additional psychological support by appropriate psychiatrists, clinical psychologists, social workers and/or other health workers. This association has also been put forward by a variety of 'fringe' medicine practitioners to justify their treatment practices.

Can cancer be prevented?

There is no known way of making any individual immune to cancer. However, it is obvious that the risk of many cancers can be considerably reduced by taking certain precautions and avoiding carcinogenic influences.

The most obvious preventive measure in reducing the risk of serious cancer is to avoid smoking. By not smoking, the risk of developing many cancers is greatly reduced, including lung cancer (eight to 10 times), mouth and throat cancer (six times), cancers of the oesophagus, stomach, pancreas and even the breast. Passive smoking (spending frequent long periods in a smoky atmosphere) is also associated with increased cancer risk and should be avoided.

The risk of the common skin cancers (basal cell carcinoma and squamous cell carcinoma) can be greatly reduced by avoiding unnecessary direct exposure to sunshine or ultra-violet light. Nature's protection is pigment in the skin in coloured races, but for fair-skinned people protective clothing such as long-sleeved shirts and wide-brimmed hats and ultraviolet-filtering skin lotions offer considerable protection. The same measures may help to some extent in avoiding melanoma, although the direct effect of sunshine on exposed skin as a cause of melanoma is less clear. It seems that to help avoid melanoma intermittent episodes of sunburn should be avoided, especially in childhood.

Diets high in fibre, including cereals, fresh fruit and vegetables and low in meat, animal fat, highly refined foods and chemically preserved foods, offer some protection against the development of stomach and bowel cancers.

The addition of iodine to the diet (usually as iodised salt) in iodine-deficient goitre belt areas may reduce the incidence of goitre and possibly of thyroid cancer. There is also some evidence that deficiency in the diet of the element selenium might predispose to some cancers (e.g. breast, bowel or prostate cancers).

Encouragement of breastfeeding may possibly be helpful in reducing the incidence of breast cancer.

Industrial laws that protect workers from a number of known industrial cancer-causing agents play a significant role in cancer prevention.

Treatment of any longstanding ulcers or chronically inflamed or irritated lesions may also be a protective measure against the development of cancer. This may affect such a variety of lesions as longstanding varicose ulcers; ulcers in the mouth possibly irritated by a jagged tooth or ill-fitting denture; gastric ulcers; ulcerative colitis of the colon or rectum; longstanding gallstones, kidney or bladder stones; chronically discharging osteomyelitis; or prolonged irritation of a pigmented lesion on the skin.

Another preventive measure is to remove or otherwise properly treat other known pre-malignant conditions such as polyps, papillomas, hyperkeratotic skin lesions, leukoplakia in the mouth or moles that show any sign of irritation or change. Also removal of benign tumours that show any evidence of enlarging or which are known to have a risk of malignant change will reduce the danger of cancer developing. Such tumours might include adenomas in the parotid gland or thyroid gland, papillomas or adenomas in the breast, cysts in the ovary, papillomas or polyps in the colon, rectum or uterus, papillomas in the bladder, or enlarging soft tissue tumours of fat (lipomas), nerve tissue (neuromas), muscle (myomas), tumours of blood or lymph vessels (haemangiomas or lymphangiomas) occasionally of cartilage (chrondromas) or bone (osteomas).

People affected by familial polyposis coli will all eventually develop colon cancer if they live to middle age, and this can be completely prevented by total removal of the colon and rectum in those people before cancer has developed.

Tests and treatments for cancer

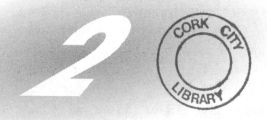

What are the symptoms of cancer?

Symptoms are complaints that cause a person to seek medical attention. Although it is true that a cancer may be present for some time before it causes symptoms, in most cases the earlier a patient seeks medical attention the better the chance of curing the cancer.

Symptoms may result from two effects of a cancer – the local effects of the cancer itself or the more general effects of the cancer as it affects the person as a whole. Usually local effects are noticed first. These might include one or more of the following: a lump; an ulcer that does not heal; pain; abnormal bleeding from the bowel, bladder, vagina or elsewhere; or interference of function of the organ or tissue involved. Such functional interference may be obstruction of the bowel in the case of bowel cancer or a persistent cough or interference with breathing in the case of lung cancer. These symptoms of local trouble will thus depend on the position of the cancer, the organ or tissue in which it started, the type of cancer cells that have developed, the size of the tumour, and the possible involvement of other organs or tissues near to the cancer.

The main general effects that may be noticed by a person with cancer are lassitude and loss of energy, loss of appetite, weight loss, the effects of blood loss or the effects of any spread of the cancer from where it started (primary site) to another organ or tissue (secondary site).

General symptoms may result not only from damage to or interference with function of the organ or tissue involved, but also from the body's reaction to the presence of cancer.

These features will be mentioned in more detail in Section 3, but some general features are outlined below.

A **lump**, **swelling** or **tumour** of some kind is present in virtually every cancer. The lump may be obvious if it is in the skin, the mouth or tongue, the breast, in lymph nodes under the skin, in fat or muscles (soft tissue), or can be felt on bone. On the other hand, not all lumps are malignant – in fact, most are not malignant – but if a new abnormal lump is found anywhere in the body it is important to seek medical advice. The most common symptom of breast cancer, for example, is a lump in the breast. The lump is often felt in the bath or shower as they are more easily felt with soapy wet hands. (Women should carry out regular monthly self-examination of the breasts, and this is best done sitting or lying in the bath using wet soapy fingers.)

An **ulcer** on the skin that does not heal quickly may be a cancer and should be examined by a doctor. Skin ulcers are usually obvious, but ulcers in the mouth or throat may be less obvious if they are painless. Any such ulcer should be examined by a doctor, especially if it has been present for more than a week or two with no evidence of healing. Most longstanding ulcers are not malignant: they may be caused by such conditions as varicose veins or poor arteries in the lower legs; or by jagged teeth, ill-fitting dentures or infections in the mouth. If there is any doubt, a doctor will arrange a biopsy. In a biopsy, a small piece of tissue is taken, usually from the edge of the ulcer, and examined under a microscope to determine its type and its cause.

Pain is usually not present early in a cancer. Most cancers are painless early in the disease. Pain usually develops only after a tumour has become big enough to press on and damage surrounding tissues or nerves. In general, a small painless lump is more likely to be a cancer than a small painful lump, and it is not advisable to wait for pain to develop before seeking medical advice.

Bleeding may be a feature of many cancers of surface tissues. For some internal cancers in the stomach, bowel, kidney, bladder, uterus or lung, bleeding is often the earliest feature. Any evidence of abnormal bleeding should be investigated. For example, with bleeding from the bowel, the blood might be bright red in colour (fresh blood) or it might be dark red or black (due to bleeding in the bowel some time previously). There may be blood in the urine; the vagina (especially between periods or after menopause); in the sputum (either from the mouth or throat or from the lung after coughing); from a mole on the skin; or from a nipple. Although bleeding may be an indication of cancer, it does not always indicate cancer, as there are many other causes of bleeding. Bleeding or bruising at several sites or small haemorrhagic spots in the skin (petechial spots) may be an indication of a blood disorder including those caused by leukaemias or lymphomas.

There may be **interference with tissue or organ function**. These symptoms vary a great deal depending on the site of a cancer. For example, a cancer in the mouth may make speaking or swallowing difficult. A cancer of the larynx will usually cause hoarseness or a change in voice. A cancer of the oesophagus is usually first noticed when there is difficulty with swallowing. A cancer of the stomach may cause difficulty with eating, change in appetite or vomiting, and a cancer of the bowel may cause a change in bowel habits (diarrhoea or constipation) or obstruct the bowel, causing bowel colic with constipation and possibly vomiting.

Cancer of the prostate may interfere with passing urine and cancer of the bladder may also cause difficulty with or frequency of passing urine.

Cancer of the lung may cause a persistent cough, local obstruction of air passages or local pneumonia, and cancers of the liver, bile ducts or pancreas may block the flow of bile from the liver, causing jaundice.

There are many other causes of these symptoms, but if any of these symptoms are noticed for the first time in someone who was otherwise well, and especially if the symptoms persist, they should be investigated.

SYMPTOMS OF SECONDARY CANCER

These symptoms will vary with the tissues or organs to which the cancer has spread.

The most common site of spread is to nearby draining **lymph nodes** in the neck, armpits, groin or elsewhere. Enlargement of these nodes may sometimes be the first feature of the presence of a cancer nearby.

Spread of cancer to the **liver** may cause jaundice or pain and swelling in the upper abdomen under the ribs on the right side. It may also lead to malnutrition, wasting and weight loss, or fluid collecting and possibly filling the abdominal cavity.

Spread of cancer to the **lungs** may cause coughing, difficulty with breathing, fever, pneumonia or chest pain.

Spread of cancer to **bones** may cause pain or fracture in the bones. It may also cause anaemia due to destruction of the blood-forming bone marrow tissues.

Spread of cancer to other soft tissues such as **fat** and **muscles** may cause swelling or lumps that may be felt under the skin.

Spread to the **bowel** or elsewhere in the abdominal cavity may cause bowel obstruction or swelling and fluid in the abdominal cavity.

Spread of cancer to the **brain** may cause severe headaches, vomiting, blurred vision, fits or unconsciousness.

Signs of cancer

The abnormalities associated with cancer may have been noticed by the patient, in which case they are called **symptoms**. If they have not been noticed by the patient but found by the doctor, they are called **signs**. The doctor therefore looks for any of those features that may not have been noticed by the patient.

The doctor looks for local lumps or other abnormal swellings, ulcers, tender or painful areas, evidence of blood loss from bowel, urine, uterus, etc. and general effects on the patient such as weight loss, and general state of health. He or she also looks for evidence of spread to other organs or tissues, knowing the likely sites for spread from any particular type of cancer. Different cancers tend to spread to different organs or tissues.

The doctor knows features of **lumps** that are most likely to be associated with cancer in general and particular forms of cancer. For example, cancer lumps are usually harder than lumps from other causes. Cancer lumps usually are not cystic (although on occasions they may be) and they are usually not tender unless quite advanced. As they enlarge, cancer lumps become adherent to nearby structures and therefore become less movable.

Cancer **ulcers** often have raised or heaped up edges. They tend to grow into other tissues on which they lie and there is usually surrounding swelling. They may bleed easily but usually not profusely. They may or may not be tender. Ulcers due to skin cancer are usually not tender, whereas malignant ulcers in the mouth and throat usually become quite tender in the later stages.

The doctor will also look for **evidence of blood loss** in the case of cancers in which bleeding is a likely feature. Blood in the faeces may be detected chemically even when it is not obvious to the naked eye (occult blood) and this may be an early feature of cancer of the stomach or bowel. In fact, occult blood loss is often used as a screening test for people with a high risk of developing gastric or bowel cancer even though they have no symptoms.

Blood in the urine may sometimes be found on microscopic examination when it is not obvious to the naked eye. This may be a feature of cancer of the kidney or bladder, although there are also other more common causes. The doctor will also carry out a general check for evidence of anaemia due to chronic blood loss.

In looking for evidence of secondary spread of cancer, the doctor will first examine the draining **lymph node** areas. For example, if a cancer in the head, mouth or throat region is suspected, the lymph nodes in the neck will be examined first. If breast cancer or cancer of the skin of the arm or chest wall is suspected, the lymph nodes in the armpits will be examined. If cancer in the lower limb or of the skin of the abdomen or lower back, scrotum, anus or vulva is suspected, the lymph nodes in the groins will be first examined.

Abdominal lymph nodes may be involved from cancers of the stomach, bowel, testes, uterus, ovaries or elsewhere in the abdominal cavity, but these are usually not able to be felt unless very large. Sometimes lymphatic channels allow tumours to spread from the abdominal organs to the lymph nodes in the neck (usually the left side); these will be examined as they are easily felt if enlarged.

Lymph nodes in the chest may be involved from cancers of the lung or the oesophagus and although these cannot be felt with the hands, evidence of their enlargement may sometimes be seen in a chest X-ray.

Lymph nodes may also be enlarged in malignant tumours known as the lymphomas or leukaemias. If enlarged, these lymph nodes are usually somewhat rubbery, and softer than nodes invaded by other cancers. They are also more likely to be smoother in outline, less likely to become fixed to other structures and often lymph nodes on both sides of the neck or lymph nodes in other places may be involved. The spleen, which is an organ in the abdomen under the ribs on the left side, also behaves like a large lymph node, and although a normal spleen cannot be felt, it may become enlarged and palpable (easily felt) in these conditions.

The doctor will also look for **evidence of lumps or swellings** in other parts of the body and especially in the abdomen, the liver or other tissues or organs likely to be involved with any cancer.

Part of the examination of the alimentary (digestive) tract would be an examination of the mouth, tongue and throat and especially an examination of the anus. Most cancers of the rectum can be felt with a gloved finger in the rectum, and many other conditions such as enlarged prostate, enlarged uterus or tumour in the pelvis can be felt by this simple examination. Also, the colour and nature of the faeces and presence of blood in the faeces can often be detected from this examination.

Which tests help in detecting cancer?

A large range of tests are now available to help detect cancer. Some of the most useful of these have become available only during the past 10 years or so and range from screening tests that

may help detect cancer in people at risk without any symptoms, to organ imaging tests in which X-rays, CT scans, ultrasound, isotope scans, MRI scans and similar investigations
including the most recent PET scans, may reveal the presence of
deep-seated tumours. There are also endoscopic tests in which
flexible mirrored tubes allow doctors to look at, photograph and
even biopsy lesions in the alimentary (digestive) tract or in other
body cavities. A number of blood and serum tests may reveal
evidence of tumour reactions somewhere in the body. However,
the most reliable investigation is the biopsy, in which a piece of
tissue is examined under a microscope to determine whether or
not a lesion contains malignant cells. The microscopic examination can very often also tell the type of malignant cells and the
organ or tissue from which they originally developed.

COMMON SCREENING TESTS
The cervical smear or 'Pap' test

One of the first and still one of the most useful specific screening
tests is the Papanicolaou or cervical smear test for detecting
early cancer at the entrance of the womb (the cervix of the
uterus). Cancer of the cervix of the uterus is the most common
form of cancer of the uterus. Women over the age of 40 years
who have had several pregnancies are most at risk from this
type of cancer, and many women now have a cervical smear test
every year. This has the advantage of being simple, painless,
cheap and relatively reliable. In this test a swab or scraping is
taken through the vagina of the entrance to the womb (or cervix
uteri). Fluid from the swab or scraping is smeared over a glass
slide and the slide is examined for cells. If malignant cells are
found, cancer may be detected early and treated with good
results. Other abnormal cells may suggest changes that could go
on to become cancer if not treated; simple treatment at that
stage can prevent a cancer developing.

Breast screening

Cancer of the breast is the most common form of serious cancer in women in most Western societies. Although there is no one completely reliable screening test, a number of tests may be combined to detect early breast cancer. These include self-examination, examination for lumps in screening clinics by a doctor or specially trained nurse, mammography (special breast X-rays), ultrasound studies and biopsy using a fine needle to suck out fluid or cells from any suspicious lump and examining the material sucked out under a microscope.

Occult blood tests

A number of chemical and other tests have been used to detect the presence of blood in the faeces where blood cannot be seen with the naked eye. The presence of blood in the faeces may indicate some abnormality in the stomach or bowel, and that abnormality may be a cancer or a pre-cancerous condition such as a polyp. This test is not always accurate, but is sometimes used as a screening test to examine people who are most at risk of cancer and to detect those most in need of further tests.

ORGAN IMAGING TESTS
X-rays

Radiological studies or X-rays are a relatively old but useful method of medical examination for cancer. Techniques are constantly improving and the doses of X-rays needed are becoming less and less. X-ray films are only able to detect spots or lesions that are different from the normal tissue in the region. This difference is seen as a relatively light or relatively dark shadow on a film. For example, X-rays pass easily through air in the lungs or gas in the large bowel, and this is shown as a dark shadow on a film. If a tumour is present in a chest X-ray, it might show as a relatively lighter or whiter part in the area normally showing as dark shadow from the air-filled lungs. On the other hand, X-rays are blocked by dense bone, which shows as a white area on film. If a tumour is present in bone, it may show as relatively dark or grey areas in the bone, which is otherwise white. Other tissues like muscle and fat are intermediate between the dark shadow of air or the white shadow of bone in their penetration by X-rays. These tissues are of similar consistency and have similar penetration by X-rays as do tumours, so that it is not so easy to detect tumour shadows in soft tissues by this method: more sophisticated investigations may be required.

Barium, iodine compounds and some other materials (often called dyes) are not penetrated by X-rays, and these are often used in the body to outline cavities that are otherwise not easily seen on an X-ray film. After a patient swallows a barium mixture (a barium meal) the dye will outline the shape of the stomach on an X-ray; if a cancer is present it may show as an abnormality in the shape or in the outline of the stomach. Similarly, a barium enema in the lower bowel may allow detection by X-rays of a cancer in the colon or rectum.

An intravenous pyelogram (IVP) or excretory urogram involves the injection of iodine compounds into a vein. When these are excreted in the urine they show on an X-ray the position, shape, size and outline of the kidneys or bladder. Iodine compounds can also be injected into the bladder or the kidneys from below (through the urine pathway), and X-rays taken. Such X-ray studies of the kidneys are called retrograde pyelograms or retrograde urograms. This test can also be used for other body cavities such as the fluid-filled space around the spinal cord; an X-ray (called a myelogram) may show an abnormal outline if a tumour is present.

Some iodine compounds are also excreted in bile into the gall bladder and bile ducts. X-rays can then be used to outline the shape and contents of the gall bladder (cholecystogram) and bile ducts (cholangiogram) which again may show abnormalities if tumours or other defects, such as gallstones, are present.

Screening

Whereas all X-rays were once recorded on a film as still photographs, techniques used now allow the radiologist to study on a television screen the movement of a radio-opaque material (dye) such as barium or iodine in a body cavity. After a barium meal or barium enema the patient is taken into a dark screening room where the radiologist can change the position of the patient to allow the material to flow into various parts of the organ being examined and more accurately determine its size, shape, position and outline on the television screen. This way the radiologist can see if a lump in the bowel, for example, is a lump of faeces that can be moved through the bowel or if it is a lump of tumour attached to the bowel wall.

Air, too, can be used to replace fluid in certain cavities and show up as shadows in X-rays. Air is sometimes used in the large bowel together with barium: the barium adheres to the wall of the bowel and the air fills the bowel cavity, allowing X-rays to show more precisely the shape of the wall of the bowel and any lump projecting into the cavity. A similar technique can be used in the cavities (ventricles) of the brain to detect evidence of some lesions. This study is known as an air encephalogram.

In most cases, the X-ray density of a cancer is similar to the X-ray density of surrounding tissues and X-ray films alone are unlikely to show evidence of a deep-seated cancer. For cancers that are not so deep-seated, however, such as breast cancer, X-rays (mammograms) may be used to detect any small differences in penetration of the tissues that may indicate the presence of a cancer.

Chest X-ray

Chest X-rays are most useful investigations for detecting abnormalities in the lungs. Abnormalities in the lungs, including tumours, may show as white opacities in the dark air-filled lungs, or the size and shape of the lungs or tissues between the lungs may be altered in size and shape. Lymph nodes in the chest are grouped around the midline between the lungs. If lymph nodes are enlarged as in the lymphomas, the centre area of white density in a chest X-ray may be widened.

Skeletal X-rays

These will show the outline and density of bones. Primary cancer of bone (i.e. cancer starting in the bone, called osteosarcoma) may sometimes be seen as an abnormal shape and abnormal density of one part of the bone, usually towards one or other end of a long bone. Secondary cancers in bone usually show as rounded, less dense areas in the bone or even as fractures. Some secondary cancers containing calcium may even show as rounded areas of increased density in the bone. However, X-rays are not infallible and will not always detect cancerous lesions in bone, especially if the lesions are small.

Mammograms

A mammogram is a special X-ray of the breast that may show the presence of cysts, dense fibrous tissue, or a cancer in the less dense fatty tissue of the breast. Small amounts of X-rays only are needed, so this examination is safe if not used excessively and may be useful as an aid to detecting breast cancer.

Angiography

Radio-opaque material (dye) may also be injected into arteries or veins or even lymph vessels for films to be taken or for immediate viewing on a television screen. The radiologist can then determine whether the vessels are in their normal position or whether they may have been pushed aside by a lump of some sort that may sometimes be a cancer. Some cancers also develop a distinctive blood supply that may also be detected by this technique. Newer methods for angiography of arteries (arteriography) have allowed arteries in virtually every part of the body to be outlined by radiographic (X-ray) techniques. These methods may be helpful in detecting evidence of deep-seated tumours that are relatively inaccessible to most other methods of investigation. Lymphangiography, by injecting radio-opaque dyes into lymph vessels, will also allow X-rays of the lymph nodes to be taken to determine whether they are enlarged or partly replaced by abnormal tissue that may be a tumour.

Isotope scans

Isotope scans (or nuclear scintigraphy) have some similarity to X-rays in that the shadows of a radioactive source are recorded on a film plate. In this case the radioactive material is injected into a vein and distributed in the bloodstream. The radioactive dose used is very small, and is made up of, or combined with, various agents depending on which organ or tissue is to be examined. Radioactive iodine, for example, is concentrated in the thyroid gland and the amount of uptake, size, shape, position, and consistency of tissue in the thyroid gland can be determined from such a test. Another such material is concentrated in bone, particularly in areas of the bone with cellular activity or growth. Thus a bone scan will not only outline the position, size and shape of bone but will also show areas of abnormal cellular activity that may be due to cancer.

Similar scans are used to outline the size, shape and any abnormal activity in the liver and spleen. In these organs, cancer may show up as one or more areas of decreased activity.

Similar radio-isotope scan tests are now available for a number of other organs or tissues including the brain, lungs and lymph nodes.

Scanning is carried out with the patient lying on a special table. Apart from a needle prick to inject the material into a vein, it is a quite painless procedure.

CT scan or CAT scan

In the early 1970s British workers developed a technique in which small doses of X-rays were used to allow the build-up of a picture of tissues in cross-section of the trunk, the head and neck or the limbs. By taking many cross-sectional pictures of the abdomen, for example, a three-dimensional concept can be developed in which the position, size and shape of all the organs, major blood vessels, bones and muscles in the abdomen can be seen and the position, size and density of any abnormal tumour or swelling assessed with considerable accuracy. CT scanning (computerised axial tomography) requires highly specialised equipment and skilled personnel and is therefore relatively expensive. Although not an infallible investigation, it has proved to be of great value in investigating many cancers and tumours in otherwise inaccessible areas of the head, abdomen, chest or deep in the limbs.

CT scanning is carried out with the patient lying on a table and, like other types of X-rays, presents no discomfort to the patient except that of lying still for several minutes on a small foam mattress in a small confined space or chamber.

Ultrasound scans

X-rays, nuclear scans and CT scans all depend on the use of small doses of penetrating X-rays or gamma rays. Although these are safe if used with proper care, there are occasions when even these small doses are probably better avoided, particularly during pregnancy, as the developing foetus is highly sensitive to irradiation. It is preferable not to expose the reproductive organs of those of child-bearing age to X-rays.

In recent years, a technique using ultrasound waves has been developed to give a somewhat similar cross-sectional picture of body tissues and organs as does the CT scan. The principle depends on sound waves being reflected or bounced back in different degrees by body tissues of different density somewhat like a radar or a depth sounder. The ultrasound waves are quite harmless.

Ultrasound scans in general do not give as much information as CT scans, but are more accurate in showing the position and type of some lesions. They may be used as an alternative to CT scans in some situations or in conjunction with CT scans in others.

Ultrasound examinations are quite painless and cause the patient no discomfort. They are safe to use in pregnancy.

MRI

MRI (magnetic resonance imaging) is a study that shows tissues on a cross-sectional film picture. Although it is similar in appearance to the CT scan, it is based on quite different principles of physics. In some parts of the body and in some body tissues such as in bone and in the brain and cranial cavity (skull box) an MRI scan may show more detail and more information than a CT scan. Sometimes both studies are used and together they may complement each other in giving slightly different information about the size, shape and other characteristics of a tumour and its extent of spread in surrounding tissues. As with CT scanning, the patient feels no pain, but is required to lie still on a firm table and in a confined space for several minutes.

PET

The PET (positron emission tomography) scan is the most recent of all non-invasive studies (studies that do not require an instrument to be put inside the body, a piece of tissue removed or a surgical operation). At the time of writing this remarkable but very costly equipment is available only in a small number of centres where intense research studies are being carried out to determine exactly how it can help in the diagnosis and treatment of cancers and other serious medical conditions.

PET scans are quite different from X-rays, CT or MRI studies. X-rays are used to produce films that show as black/white shadows with shades of grey. These are inexpensive and readily available, but do not give nearly as much information as CT or MRI films. Both CT and MRI scans give more three-dimensional information about the position, size, shape and consistency of tumours or lumps deep to the surface and their position in relation to other tissues like arteries, nerves, muscles, bone and important organs. They are also produced in black and white pictures with shades of grey. They are based on laws of physics using penetration of X-rays and other rays under different conditions, including a change in magnetic fields in the case of MRI.

Although PET scans produce three-dimensional pictures that may be in black and white or in colour, they are based on different chemical activity in different types of tissues and different cells. The basic principle is that cancer cells use more glucose than normal cells: PET scans show areas of different glucose activity in body tissues. PET scans are often able to show something of the activity of the cancer such as its rate of growth and any changes made to the cancer by treatment given. For some cancers they are better able to show whether the cancer has spread to other places. They may also indicate whether a cancer has responded to treatment or whether it might be starting to come back again after treatment.

PET scanning is a very safe study but it is expensive. As its real place in investigation and treatment of cancer is not yet known, many more studies must be made and costs contained before it can be made more widely available.

ENDOSCOPIC EXAMINATIONS

Most people are familiar with a dentist using a mirror to examine the back of the teeth and a doctor using a head mirror to reflect light waves into the mouth to examine the throat, larynx, or back of the nose. In recent years, the principle of using mirrors and lenses with a light source to examine the inside of body cavities has been refined to degrees of precision not considered feasible a decade or two ago. Previously, non-operative examination of the inside of body cavities was limited to examination of the larynx, trachea and air passages (bronchi), oesophagus, stomach, rectum and lower large bowel, bladder and vagina through rigid or semi-rigid tubes. These are still useful methods of examination, as they allow ready examination of these organs. They are reasonably simple to use, reasonably cheap to buy and are readily available either in doctors' surgeries or in hospitals.

Sigmoidoscopy

Although largely replaced by a more flexible colonoscope, a sigmoidoscope can still allow a valuable examination for large bowel cancer. About 50% of all large bowel cancers are within reach of a rigid sigmoidoscope. Sigmoidoscopy can be done in a doctor's surgery without anaesthesia, and a biopsy of any suspicious tissue can be taken at the time of examination. Some precautions are first taken to empty the bowel. The patient usually lies on one side and the sigmoidoscope is passed through the anus. Air is blown into the bowel to inflate it and so open up

the lumen or bowel cavity. This air and the passage of the instrument is uncomfortable but not unbearably so.

Proctoscopy

Examination of the anus and lower rectum can be carried out
quite simply in a doctor's surgery with a small metal tube-like
instrument called a proctoscope or anal speculum. Although it
does not penetrate far into the rectum, it can be useful for
detecting or treating lesions in or near the anus such as haemor-
rhoids or cancer of the anus, which is rather rare.

Vaginal speculum

A vaginal speculum is a metal instrument that allows a doctor to
examine the walls of the vagina or cervix of the uterus in the
surgery without significant discomfort to the patient.

Laryngoscopy and bronchoscopy

The larynx may be examined indirectly with a mirror in the
doctor's surgery, but a more direct examination of the sensitive
larynx or main air passages is usually carried out with a rigid
laryngoscope or bronchoscope in hospital under general anaesthesia.

Oesophagoscopy

Examinations of the oesophagus in the past have usually been
carried out in hospital under general anaesthesia using rigid
instruments.

Cystoscopy

The bladder may be examined with a rigid cystoscope, usually in
hospital under general anaesthesia.

FLEXIBLE SCOPES

Advances have been made with flexible instruments, mainly with the fibre-optic gastroscope or colonoscope, but more flexible scopes are now being developed to replace many of the rigid metal scopes previously used.

Gastroscopy

Expert gastroenterologists can pass modern gastroscopes through the patient's mouth into the stomach without general anaesthesia; provided the patient is suitably sedated, they are passed with little discomfort. Gastroscopes allow examination not only of the oesophagus and stomach, but also of the first part of the small bowel (duodenum). Through the duodenum they also allow examination of the opening of the bile duct from the liver and gall bladder and the pancreatic duct from the pancreas. Radio-opaque material can be injected into these ducts, allowing X-rays to be taken for more detailed examination.

Colonoscopy

The colonoscope is a flexible instrument that can be passed through the anus and around the whole length of large bowel to allow its examination. The instrument can be used to remove pre-malignant polyps or to take biopsies. Special preparation is required to empty the bowel before the colonoscope is used. This instrument may be passed without undue discomfort if the patient is well sedated, although some patients may prefer general anaesthesia.

Peritonoscopy (laparoscopy) and thoracoscopy

The body cavities – the peritoneal cavity of the abdomen and the thoracic or pleural cavities of the chest – may also be examined by passing instruments called a peritoneoscope or thoracoscope through a small incision into the cavity. This is carried out under general anaesthesia in the operating theatre. In some situations biopsies may be taken. Special equipment is now available to carry out some surgical operations using similar scopes with surgical instruments passed through a second small opening in the abdominal or chest wall. Even some cancer operations have been carried out in this way.

Culdoscopy

Culdoscopy is an examination of the pelvis. The instrument is passed into the pelvic cavity through a small incision made in the top of the back wall of the vagina.

BLOOD AND SERUM TESTS

Blood tests may show either direct or indirect evidence of cancer.

Haemoglobin and red cell count

Most cancers eventually cause some degree of anaemia, and haemoglobin and red blood cell counts will show evidence of this. Some tumours might be quite advanced, however, before evidence of anaemia is present.

White cell count

The white cell count may also be affected in some types of cancer. More significantly, examination of the number and type of white cells may show the first evidence of a leukaemia.

Serum biochemistry

Some types of cancer are likely to change biochemical components in the blood. For example, cancer of the prostate gland may result in an elevation of the enzyme called serum acid phosphatase; advanced breast cancer may cause elevation of serum calcium; and a particular type of large bowel cancer may cause loss of potassium from the bowel and a fall in serum potassium may result. Cancers in the liver may cause a degree of liver failure which may also be detected by changes in serum bio-chemistry.

Tumour markers

Cancer researchers have been looking for some years to find some specific component of the blood that might indicate the presence of chemical products in the blood as a result of a cancer or the body's defence reactions to a cancer. Most studies involved the study of immune reactions in the body to the presence of cancer. As yet there are not many tests of practical value available for clinical use, but the most widely used of these tests are the CEA, the alpha-feto-protein and PSA tests.

A **CEA** test is a test for the presence of CEA (carcino-embryonic antigen) in blood. The material CEA is thought to be released from some cancer cells, especially cancers of the large bowel. A high level or titre of this material may suggest the presence of bowel cancer, and a return to a low level after treatment may indicate that most or all of the cancer has been eradicated.

The **alpha-feto-protein** test is a similar test which may indicate the presence of a primary liver cancer called hepatoma.

A **PSA** test is a blood test that may indicate abnormality of the prostate gland in men. Sometimes this abnormality may be cancer of the prostate, especially if the level of PSA (prostate specific antigen) is high. A return to low levels after treatment may indicate that the cancer has been eradicated and the patient cured.

Tumour marker tests are not totally reliable, but a great deal of work is being carried out in this field. It seems certain that valuable tumour marker tests, indicating the presence or absence of specific cancers, will be available for clinical use in the not too distant future.

BIOPSY

The most reliable test for cancer is the tissue biopsy, in which a piece of tissue is taken from a suspected cancer and examined under a microscope. Provided a proper sample of tissue is taken, examination of the cells in the biopsy specimen will usually allow a pathologist to determine not only whether a cancer is present, but also the type of cancer, the tissue of origin of the cancer and even the degree of malignancy. Sometimes the biopsy may also give a good indication of the likelihood of a cure.

Biopsies are usually taken by a surgeon at operation; the surgeon will take a small representative sample of a suspected cancer (incision biopsy) or, if the tumour is small, he or she may remove the whole tumour for examination (excision biopsy).

A number of techniques have been developed to assist a diagnosis by biopsy.

For some tumours – as for example, some lumps in the breast, it may be possible to insert a special needle into the lump and aspirate or suck out sufficient cells or tissue for biopsy examination (**needle aspiration biopsy**). There is also a special needle called 'Trucut' with a mechanism that allows a small core of tissue to be punched out ('punch out' biopsy). This might be done under local anaesthesia without admission to hospital. Provided a correct specimen is taken and an expert team is available to examine it, a diagnosis can be made rapidly with little disturbance to the patient.

Needle aspiration or punch out biopsy may now be used for a number of different types of tumours in a variety of other tissues such as the prostate gland, the liver, the thyroid gland, or deep-seated tumours in the limbs or chest.

Aspiration cytology is similar to aspiration biopsy except that it also applies to the examination for cells in cysts or other fluid. A cyst in the breast or elsewhere may be aspirated and by special preparation the contents examined for the presence of malignant cells. If malignant cells are found, a diagnosis of cancer can be made. If, however, no malignant cells are found, there may still be some doubt that cancer is present. It is possible that cancer cells could be in the cyst but not in the sample of fluid taken.

In **bone marrow biopsy**, a similar aspiration technique is used to obtain specimens of bone marrow for determining the presence and type of suspected leukaemia.

Frozen section biopsy is a technique used to prepare biopsy specimens for examination. Usually, the preparation and staining of a biopsy specimen for microscopic examination takes three or four days or even longer. The tissue is prepared, embedded in a wax block, and stained in different ways to reveal special features of the cells. For some tumours it may be important for the surgeon to know the diagnosis immediately, so that any necessary cancer operation can be completed without delay. By using the technique of frozen section, in which the biopsy specimen is prepared by immediately being frozen solid and then stained, the pathologist may be able to give the surgeon an accurate diagnosis within a few minutes. If the patient is anaesthetised and prepared for operation, the surgeon may be able to completely remove the cancer at the same operation. Frozen section techniques are now highly accurate for most cancers if used by skilled pathologists, but for other cancers it may not be possible to determine an accurate diagnosis until special wax pathology sections have been prepared in the usual way.

Can cancer be cured?

Although cancer is a frightening word, it is a fact that in modern developed societies most cancers are cured. The curability of a cancer depends on the type of cancer and the tissue from which it has grown, the position of the tumour in the body, the degree of abnormality of the individual cancer cells, the size of the cancer, the structures into which it may have grown and the presence and site of any secondary spread of the cancer. The age and general health of the patient may also be of significance. The patient's natural defence reactions are probably highly significant, although as yet not clearly understood and not yet able to be measured with any degree of confidence.

Many of the most significant factors will depend on how quickly the cancer is detected and treated. A small cancer detected early and before it has spread or involved other tissues may be eminently curable, whereas the same cancer neglected, perhaps for some months, until it has enlarged and spread to other sites, may be quite incurable.

The best chance of curing cancer lies in the hands of the therapist or team of therapists who make the first attempt. That is, a cancer that has recurred after a failed attempt at treatment is more difficult to cure than it was at the first attempt. The quality of treatment given to the patient, especially in the initial treatment, is therefore a most important factor in determining whether or not a cure is likely to result.

In westernised societies, more cancers are cured than not cured simply because the most common cancers are basal cell cancers of skin and squamous cell cancers of skin. Not only do these cancers grow relatively slowly and spread relatively late, if at all, they are obvious to the patient and doctor when they are quite small, and if properly treated at that stage are eminently curable. However, even disregarding basal cell and squamous cell carcinomas, more than half of all patients with more serious cancers can now be cured. Even the more aggressive and dangerous pigmented skin cancer, the melanoma, is usually quite curable in its early stages, and with people becoming more aware of the danger of any change in a pigmented mole, or other dark spot on the skin, most melanomas are now detected and cured before they have spread.

Cancers that are least likely to be cured are often those that develop in deep body tissues and are not usually obvious until they have reached a stage when they have spread to lymph nodes or other tissues. These include cancer of the oesophagus, stomach, pancreas and lung. Hence the search for methods of early detection of these cancers. Other cancers with poor prognosis include those in organs that cannot easily be dispensed with such as the liver or brain. Until recently, cancers that develop in cells scattered widely throughout the body tissues such as the lymphomas and leukaemias were considered incurable, but with modern treatment methods, increasing numbers of patients with these malignancies are also being cured.

The common cancers of the breast, prostate and bowel and cancers of the uterus are somewhat intermediate in their prognosis. It is most important that these cancers are detected early, as the outlook is much better if treatment starts when they are small. For this reason, cancer screening clinics have been established to detect potentially curable cancers before they reach an incurable stage.

What treatments are available?

The three mainstays of cancer treatment are surgery, radiotherapy and chemotherapy.

SURGERY

Surgery is the oldest form of cancer treatment. The surgeon's objective is to excise the cancer in its entirety, together with all adjacent tissues into which cancer cells may have spread. For some types of cancer, especially for early skin cancers and small cancers in the mouth, surgery offers a relatively simple, straightforward, quick and effective treatment method. For cancers that have spread to or are likely to have spread to draining lymph nodes, the surgeon removes not only the primary cancer but all the draining lymph nodes likely to be involved. The primary cancer and lymph nodes are best removed in one block of tissue where this is feasible. If a great deal of tissue has to be removed, the surgeon may need to do some form of plastic or reconstructive procedure to leave as little defect or deformity as possible.

For breast cancer that is confined to the breast with possible early involvement of lymph nodes in the axilla (armpit), the most common surgical treatment over the past 100 years has been total removal of the affected breast and lymph nodes from the armpit as one block of tissue (radical mastectomy).

For deep-seated cancers, the whole or part of the involved organ is usually excised together with nearby draining lymph nodes. This is standard treatment for cancer of the stomach, colon, rectum, uterus, oesophagus, lung, kidney and sometimes the pancreas.

Sarcomas in limbs tend to recur unless widely excised, and often the best chance of cure by surgery, especially for big sarcomas, is by amputation of an affected limb. Newer techniques of combined treatment (see page 58) have reduced the need for amputation in many cases.

RADIOTHERAPY

Radiotherapy is the second oldest effective form of treatment for cancer in developed societies, but has been available only since the turn of the century. Treatment depends on the sensitivity of dividing cells to X-rays or gamma rays emitted from a radioactive source. Treatment, equipment and techniques are constantly being improved, with better results in eradicating cancer cells and causing less damage to surrounding tissues and cells.

Radiotherapy has the advantage of averting a surgical operation, but in many cases treatment over three, four or five weeks is required. It also has the disadvantage of causing some damage to normal tissues and cells surrounding the cancer in the area treated (irradiation field). The objective of the radiotherapist is to position the patient and the radiation fields in such a way as to include all the tumour in the radiation field, with minimal exposure of normal tissue, thus achieving greatest destruction of tumour cells with as little as possible damage to normal tissues and cells.

Radiotherapy is effective treatment for many skin, mouth and throat cancers and for some deep-seated cancers that cannot be totally removed by surgery. It is also used as a palliative treatment to reduce the size of some cancers that cannot be cured by other means.

The dose of radiotherapy used is critical, and must be determined by experts. Too little will not destroy cancer cells, but too much will destroy normal tissues, and may result in painful ulcers that may not heal and other long-term local problems. The dose is also cumulative, that is, once radiotherapy has been given to a part of the body in a treatment dose, it cannot ever be given again to the same site without risk of serious tissue damage.

Radiotherapy is quite painless, although it may leave some skin changes like sunburn and the patient may feel listless and tired after treatment. Although the red flush of skin change settles after a few weeks, some minor skin changes with small dilated blood vessels are often a permanent feature of an area that has been irradiated.

CHEMOTHERAPY

Doctors, scientists and others have been searching over the centuries for chemical substances that might cure cancer. The effect of some naturally occurring hormones in depressing growth of some cancers was first noticed early this century, but it was only in 1945, when it was observed that mustard gas destroyed dividing cells, that nitrogen mustard was discovered as a drug that could be used clinically against cancer cells. Many effective anti-cancer drugs have been developed since that time. These drugs have their greatest effect on dividing cells: as cancer cells divide more constantly than normal body cells, they are more likely to be affected than the normal cells. The present anti-cancer drugs are grouped or classified according to the manner in which they affect dividing cells. In treating cancers the specialist cancer clinician (oncologist) selects drugs that are known to be effective against the type of cancer being treated with least possible damage to normal body cells. In general, appropriate combinations of effective drugs are more effective than large doses of one drug only, and much research is being done to discover the most effective and safe combinations and dose and timing schedules of drugs against different types of cancer.

Palliative chemotherapy

The most widely applied use of the anti-cancer drugs is in treating widespread cancers or cancers that for one reason or another cannot be treated effectively by surgery or by radio-therapy. Although some cancers can be cured by drugs, in general this form of treatment is palliative. (Palliation means that the cancer may be reduced in size and the patient given relief of symptoms for some time, but almost invariably the cancer will recur sooner or later, and eventually death from the cancer is likely.)

Palliative chemotherapy, by reducing the cancer, will usually prolong life and make the patient more comfortable. Sometimes, however, because of the inconvenience and problems associated with treatment and the possible distress of side-effects (see page 59) there is doubt as to whether palliative chemotherapy is worthwhile. In each case the medical attendants should discuss the likely benefits and possible problems with the patient and his or her family before a final decision is made about the treatment. Although it is the doctor's responsibility to give informed advice, the final decision as to whether to have or not have palliative chemotherapy should be made by the patient. If doubt exists in the patient's mind about such treatment, a trial course of treatment may be appropriate – that is, treatment is begun with the proviso that if the patient finds it too distressing, it can be modified or stopped at any time.

Adjuvant chemotherapy

More recently, anti-cancer drugs have been used to destroy any cancer cells that may remain in the body after all obvious cancer cells have been removed, usually by surgery. Anti-cancer drugs are given after surgery in cancers where it is known there is a significant risk that scattered cancer cells may be present, even though they cannot be detected.

At present, the most appropriate use of adjuvant chemotherapy is in treating women who have had a breast cancer treated by surgery (mastectomy) and people (usually young people) who have had bone cancer (osteosarcoma) treated by surgery that may have been amputation of a limb.

Regional chemotherapy

Although surgery is limited to treating cancers localised to a particular region that can be excised and radiotherapy is limited to treating cancer cells in a limited radiation field, chemotherapy is generally given systemically, that is, to the body as a whole. Anti-cancer drugs are sometimes given by mouth or more commonly by injection into a vein. The drug is absorbed into the bloodstream and distributed by the blood to all parts of the body.

When cancers are limited to one particular region of the body and that region is supplied with blood by one particular artery, it is sometimes possible to concentrate the anti-cancer drugs on the cancer by injecting or infusing the drugs directly into the artery supplying blood to the cancer. This is called regional or intra-arterial chemotherapy.

Combined integrated treatment

For relatively small and relatively uncomplicated localised cancers that can be effectively treated by surgery or radiotherapy, these forms of treatment are best used in a straightforward and usually simple fashion.

For some cancers, however, surgery alone or radiotherapy alone may not be able to cure most patients, or a surgical operation required to eradicate the cancer may be so mutilating as to be unacceptable to the patient. In these circumstances, better results can sometimes be achieved by combining surgery and/or radiotherapy and/or chemotherapy.

Present-day treatment of some breast cancers is an example of a widely accepted use of combined treatment. For women with moderately advanced breast cancer, the breast and axillary (armpit) lymph nodes are usually removed surgically. Nearby lymph nodes that have not been removed at operation may be treated by radiotherapy, but adjuvant chemotherapy is given (by injections) to control any cancer that may have escaped in the circulation and caused growths in other organs or tissues.

Induction (neoadjuvant) chemotherapy

In treating some cancers that appear to remain localised to the site of origin but which are unlikely to be cured by surgery or radiotherapy alone, another form of combined treatment is sometimes successful. In these situations the chemotherapy is best given first to reduce the size and extent of the cancer and to reduce its ability to grow and spread. It may then be possible to totally remove the reduced tumour by either surgery or radiotherapy. If the prospects of cure by either surgery or radio-therapy are still not good, it is often possible to use both radiotherapy and surgery after the chemotherapy. Work in this form of combined treatment is showing encouraging results, especially with some cancers in the head and neck including the mouth and throat, some cancers in the stomach, some breast cancers and some cancers and sarcomas in limbs. In these situations it may be possible to give the chemotherapy more effectively by using the intra-arterial infusion technique of regional chemotherapy.

Side-effects of chemotherapy

The risk of using cytotoxic anti-cancer drugs is that as well as killing cancer cells they also cause damage to normal body cells. As with radiotherapy, the doses given and methods of adminis-tration must be arranged by experts familiar with their use so that maximum damage to cancer cells with minimum damage to normal cells and body tissues will result. Cells that are dividing are the most susceptible to these agents. Cancer cells, which are constantly dividing, are therefore more susceptible than normal cells. However, a number of cells in normal tissues divide frequently to repair and replace tissues and cells that are con-stantly being worn out or lost. These include blood-forming cells (in the bone marrow), surface skin and hair cells, cells lining the mouth, throat, stomach and bowel, and cells lining the air passages. The most serious side-effect of most anti-cancer agents is a fall in the white cells or platelets in the blood: this may lead to a reduced resistance to infection, or to bleeding. Regular blood counts are taken to determine whether the doses of drugs may need to be adjusted. Other possible side-effects are mouth and throat ulcers, nausea and vomiting, hair loss or bleeding from the bowel. While some of these side-effects are common, they are all reversible after the drugs have been stopped.

A small number of anti-cancer drugs may affect function of the heart or lungs or nerves, but these effects are not often seen as they are unlikely to occur with normal doses of drugs used. However, doctors still watch closely, and at any sign of these problems these drugs are stopped. With proper supervision by experts familiar with the use of these drugs (oncologists), the risk of serious problems is small.

Cells in the ovaries of young women and cells in the testes of men are constantly dividing to produce ova (eggs) and sperma-tozoa (sperms) for potential reproduction and new embryo production. If chemotherapy is essential in such people they are advised to avoid initiating a pregnancy during treatment and for at least 12 months afterwards due to the risk of producing abnormal ova or spermatozoa. There is even a risk of permanent sterility. In the case of men, spermatozoa can be produced and kept in cold storage (in liquid nitrogen) before chemotherapy is started so that it can be used for fertilisation at a later date. It may sometimes be possible to take and store ova from women before commencing chemotherapy. These can be fertilised and implanted into the uterus at a later date if subsequent cancer treatment has been successful.

Other important treatments

HORMONE THERAPY

In 1941 two American doctors, Charles Huggins and Clarence Hodges, showed that in a large percentage of cases, cancers of the prostate regressed either after the removal of male hormone (by castration) or by the administration of a female hormone (oestrogen). This was the first demonstration that some cancers are hormone-dependent and could respond to manipulation of certain natural body hormones. Since then some other cancers have been found to be hormone-dependent. Often these can be influenced by giving the patient an antagonistic hormone. That is, a cancer that is stimulated or dependent on a particular type of hormone is likely to be inhibited or suppressed by the removal of the source of that hormone or by giving a hormone that has the opposite effect. Oestrogen therapy and castration are still used as standard treatment of cancer of the prostate, with worthwhile control in the majority of patients, although the desire and ability to have sex is suppressed and other changes in sexual characteristics may occur such as enlargement of the man's breast tissue caused by oestrogen.

Breast cancer

In a number of women, especially young (pre-menopausal) women, breast cancer is, to a greater or lesser extent, dependent on the female sex hormone called oestrogen. Giving more oestrogen to these patients could cause the cancer to grow more rapidly. On the other hand, removal of the source of the patient's own body oestrogen (i.e. removal of the ovaries) results in regression of the breast cancer to a greater or lesser degree in most patients. Removal of the ovaries is therefore often used in treating cancer of the breast in young women if the cancer is widespread or so advanced that it cannot be cured by surgery or radiotherapy. Unfortunately, removal of the ovaries or other hormone treatments rarely, if ever, results in complete cure, but often results in worthwhile regression for a period.

In older women whose ovaries are not actively functioning, or in younger women who have had their ovaries removed, a further improvement may be achieved by giving male hormones called androgens. An even greater number will respond to a more recently developed anti-oestrogen product called tamoxifen.

Although tamoxifen is the most effective and most widely used hormonal agent (actually an anti-hormone), and rarely causes any upset to the patient in the short term (over a year or two), when used over several years there is some risk that it may alter and even stimulate a cancer in the uterus. This risk is quite small, but most doctors now limit the use of tamoxifen to two years or so unless it is essential to use it for longer periods.

Manipulation of hormones, and especially the use of tamoxifen, has a distinct advantage over other forms of chemotherapy, as hormones are less likely to cause prolonged nausea and other serious side-effects. However, the male hormone, androgen, will cause most female patients to develop certain male characteristics such as a deepening of the voice and growth of hair on the face. It may also cause an increase in sexual desire which can be distressing for some patients. Modified androgens with reduced side-effects are an improvement, but none is entirely without side-effects.

Another form of hormone therapy is to remove or otherwise put out of action other glands that are responsible for oestrogen production after the ovaries have ceased to function or have been removed. These glands are the adrenal glands which are just above the kidneys, or the pituitary gland at the base of the brain just above the back of the nose. Either the adrenal or the pituitary gland can be removed surgically, or their actions suppressed by the use of certain drugs. If this is done, other precautions must be taken and medications given to replace other essential functions of these glands.

The more recently developed anti-oestrogen compound tamoxifen has a similar effect to androgen but has the advantage of being almost free of side-effects. Tamoxifen is also more likely to be effective in a larger number of patients, including older women, than androgens or other agents.

Not all breast cancers will respond to hormone therapy.

When a breast cancer biopsy is taken, a small piece is usually tested for hormone sensitivity (called the oestrogen and progesterone receptor tests). These tests will give an indication as to whether the cancer is likely to respond to hormone manipulation. If not, then some other form of treatment such as cytotoxic chemotherapy may be used.

The adrenal gland hormone, cortisone, may also have the effect of suppressing some cancers and is often used in combination with cytotoxic chemotherapeutic drugs in treatment of breast cancer, some cases of leukaemia, the lymphomas, especially Hodgkin's disease, adenocarcinoma of the kidney, and a rare cancer of bone marrow called multiple myeloma.

Other cancers that respond to hormones include cancer in the male breast, which will often respond to castration, and cancer of the lining inside the womb (endometrial cancer of the uterus), which may respond to the hormone progesterone. Sometimes cancer of the kidney will respond either to male or female hormones, and occasionally thyroid cancer will be suppressed by the use of the thyroid hormone, thyroxin.

Hormone side-effects

Hormone therapy has the advantage of being well tolerated by most patients and relatively free of serious side-effects in comparison to cytotoxic chemotherapeutic drugs. However, hormones may sometimes have some serious side-effects. Oestrogens in males may cause thrombosis and some feminising effects and androgens in females may cause high blood pressure as well as masculinising effects. Removal of the adrenals or pituitary glands also leaves problems of endocrine balance that must be managed.

Hormone treatment is often more readily accepted by patients and the medical profession as being more natural, more scientific and less toxic than cytotoxic chemotherapy. Unfortunately, however, the good responses of hormone treatment are usually relatively short-lived and eventually the cancers re-develop. Each time they redevelop they are less responsive to other forms of hormone management and eventually become unaffected by all forms of hormone management.

IMMUNOTHERAPY

The body's natural defence against invasion by organisms and other foreign matter is through its immune defence system. There is a good deal of evidence that the body also has immune defences against malignant cells, and the development of cancer is possibly due to some fault or breakdown in these protective mechanisms.

Much research is concerned with determining the nature of these immunological defence mechanisms and trying to improve or assist them. Although there is hope that these approaches will one day be of considerable practical value in the treatment of cancer, at the present stage there is little to offer in the way of effective practical treatment.

Injections of certain relatively harmless organisms such as the cowpox virus BCG (a harmless bacterium) or *Corynebacterium parvum* (another harmless bacterium) have been used in trials in the treatment of some malignancies to stimulate natural immune defence mechanisms. Some isolated successes have been reported with these and other 'immune' preparations, especially in the treatment of melanoma and lymphomas, but as yet consistent clinical benefit has not been found and for most cancers little if any benefit has resulted.

New immune preparations are constantly under study, but three groups of immunological substances of particular interest are the interferons, the interleukins and tumour necrosis factor (TNF).

Interferon

It was first recognised in the 1930s that infection of animal cells with one virus would for a time 'interfere' with infection by other viruses. Thirty years later it was discovered that a protein substance was released from cells infected with a virus and this substance protected other cells against other viral infections. This interfering substance is called interferon.

Interferon is found to be species specific. That is, interferon produced by chicken cells is protective of other chicken cells against virus infection but does not give similar protection in any other animal. Similarly, interferon produced from human cells is protective for other human cells but not for cells of other animal species.

Because it is difficult and expensive to prepare large quantities of interferon, trials to study its clinical value in large numbers of patients have been difficult to arrange. There is evidence that it may be protective in viral infections but is too expensive for general use. Some tumours possibly associated with virus infection (e.g. osteogenic sarcoma of bone) have been investigated, and although some encouraging early results were reported, long-term good results have not been maintained.

The condition AIDS (acquired immune deficiency syndrome) is caused by virus infection. This condition is an infection and not a cancer, but it can result in the development of a particular type of cancer called Karposi's sarcoma. Early hope that AIDS might respond to interferon treatment or any other immune treatment has so far not been fulfilled.

The interleukins

The interleukins are protein substances produced from white cells and are found to activate the immunological defence system. The first interleukins were Interleukin I, which is produced from macrophages (giant white cells) and Interleukin II, which is produced from lymphocytes (small white cells). They stimulate reproduction and activity of immune cells against a cancer to which the cells have been specifically sensitised. In experimental animals, interleukins have been shown under certain conditions to so stimulate the animal's natural lymphocyte activity against implanted cancers that the cancers have been completely eradicated. However, at the time of writing, neither Interleukin I nor Interleukin II nor several other more recently discovered interleukins have made any major impact on cancer treatment.

TNF

TNF (tumour necrosis factor) is a more recent product of immunological research. This product does cause cancer cell destruction in some experimental models, but is too toxic for direct use in human patients. Recent work in Europe has shown, however, that TNF enhances the anti-cancer effect of certain other chemotherapeutic agents and can be used safely and effectively when given to a part of the body only. At the time of writing, it can only be given with safety in a closed circuit by regional perfusion or regional infusion to treat malignancies such as melanoma and sarcoma when confined to a limb (see *Regional chemotherapy*, p 57).

Some treatments under study

HEAT THERAPY

It is well known that cancer cells are more sensitive to heat than are normal cells. A number of researchers and clinicians have been investigating methods of applying localised heat to organs or tissues containing cancer in a manner that will safely destroy the cancer cells but not damage the normal body tissues. This approach could be particularly valuable for treating cancer cells in a vital organ that cannot be safely removed such as the liver. Several types of microwave-emitting machines have been designed for this purpose. A number of problems have yet to be solved, particularly in maintaining the heat at a critical level for a significant period without overheating the patient or causing damage to normal tissues and cells. However, after several years of study the most that can be said is that some interesting and hopeful results have been reported.

Heat therapy is also being studied in conjunction with chemotherapy in treating some tumours confined to a limb, e.g. melanoma. There is no doubt that when the chemotherapy and heat can be confined to the limb circulation there is a greater tumour response than when chemotherapy alone is used. However, with this combined treatment there is also more risk of damage to normal muscles, skin and other tissues in the limb.

LASER SURGERY

Laser surgery is simply a development of surgical technique in cancer treatment in which a laser is used to cut tissues or to destroy tumour tissue that is exposed to the laser light.

CRYOSURGERY

This is another technique of destroying tumour tissue by using an extremely cold temperature application to freeze-thaw and so destroy the tissue. It has been used for years to treat small skin pre-malignant lesions (dry ice or liquid nitrogen) but recently a probe has been developed to destroy secondary deposits of cancer cells, especially in the liver.

PHOTODYNAMIC THERAPY

This is a new type of treatment being investigated for some cancers.

The small new capillary blood vessels that develop with a cancer to supply it with blood are poorly formed and fragile. They easily break down if damaged and also allow some chemicals to leak out into the cancer tissues. Photodynamic therapy depends on a technique of giving the patients certain photosensitive chemical substances by intravenous injection. These substances leak out of the fragile blood vessels in the cancer and the cancer is then subjected to laser light of certain wavelengths. The reaction of the substances to laser light destroys the cancer cells. As laser light does not penetrate any distance into tissues, this treatment is only used at this stage to treat certain surface cancers such as in the mucous membrane lining the mouth. Studies to date are being carried out only in highly specialised clinics as precautions must be taken to avoid side-effects, especially general sunlight hypersensitivity.

Advantages of this treatment over other more standard treatments are as yet uncertain, but in the future there may be potential for developing similar techniques to treat other less accessible cancers.

Care of general health

The presence of cancer in the body sooner or later will have a profound effect on the patient's general state of health. Anorexia (loss of appetite), weight loss, anaemia, lassitude and general debility are common general features, and specific problems will develop according to the site of the cancer and the tissues or organs involved. The ability of the body's natural defence mechanisms to control cancer will be affected by the patient's general state of health, mental and emotional state and ability to tolerate the various forms of treatment.

For these reasons, it is important that special attention be paid to the patient's general health. The diet should be nutritious yet tempting and interesting. Adequate vitamins must be provided either in the food or with vitamin supplements. Any anaemia should be appropriately treated and there should be provision for adequate rest and gentle healthy exercise. There must be adequate provision for pain relief.

Treatment of complications, and palliative care

Special problems associated with particular forms of cancer will need appropriate attention. This may include attention to nutrition for patients with obstructive cancer of oesophagus or stomach; relief of obstruction for patients with bowel cancer; or pancreatic cancer obstructing the bile duct and causing jaundice; relief of urinary obstruction in cancer of the prostate gland; and adequate local treatment and dressing for cancers fungating through the skin. Pressure on the lungs with breathlessness caused by fluid accumulated around the lungs in the pleural cavity may be at least temporarily relieved by removing the fluid. Similarly, removal of fluid accumulated in the abdominal cavity may temporarily relieve pressure in the abdomen and lower chest.

Raised intra-cranial pressure (inside the skull) may cause headaches, vomiting, convulsions or loss of consciousness (coma). This may be caused by tumours, with surrounding swelling in the brain. The patient can often be relieved by the use of certain drugs that reduce the swelling or by radiotherapy.

Complicating infections with cancer such as pneumonia associated with cancer obstructing the air passages will also require appropriate attention.

Bones involved with cancer may not only be painful but may fracture spontaneously – a condition known as pathological fracture. Pathological fractures need to be treated on their merits, but healing is often helped by local radiotherapy. Secondary cancers not only in bones but also in liver, lungs, brain, bowel and other situations may also need special treatment.

Pain relief

Nothing is more wearing, debilitating and distressing for people than to suffer constant pain. Although most cancers causing severe pain are usually advanced and some are not curable, those suffering from severe pain can at least be given relief. For curable cancers the best pain relief is achieved by eradicating the cancer, but many pain-relieving measures are available for incurable cancers. Radiotherapy will often reduce the size of the tumour and reduce surrounding swelling and pressure, so giving pain relief. This is especially so for secondary cancers in bones and the brain. Operations to relieve obstruction of bowel, bladder or other organs will give pain relief. Hormones or anti-cancer drugs that reduce the size of tumours, thus reducing any associated pressure, may also be used on occasions to effect pain relief.

Nerves that transmit pain sensation may also be put out of action by injecting them with local anaesthetic or with alcohol, or possibly by cutting them surgically to relieve pain. Occasionally the nerve pathway in the spinal cord that conducts pain sensation to the brain can be cut to give permanent loss of pain sensation from a region of the body.

Meditation, hypnotherapy or acupuncture are sometimes used for pain relief. Although these may be helpful with some patients, with others their greatest value may be in emotional support rather than in relief of severe or constant pain.

The most common and quickest method of pa[...]
the use of simple pain-relieving drugs (analgesic[s])
and addictive pain-relieving drugs (narcotics). Sim[...]
such as aspirin and aspirin-like products, paracetamol (ace[...]
minophen) and the like, are usually used first. If not effective,
agents containing small amounts of the least dangerous narcotic
agent, codeine, are often used. The stronger narcotic agents,
pethidine (meperidine), methadone, and the opium derivative,
morphine, may be given for immediate relief of severe pain,
usually as a temporary measure until other treatment has given
more permanent pain relief. They may also be given on a permanent basis in cases where the cancer is incurable and the
person has a limited life expectancy. In some countries heroin is
also used very effectively in these circumstances, but only where
it is certain that life expectancy is strictly limited.

Psychotherapy and spiritual help

Some psychologists and alternative medicine practitioners as
well as some well qualified psychiatrists postulate that sometimes cancer may be a result of anxiety, emotional trauma or
depressive states. This may or may not be so, but it must at least
be recognised that such emotional states may well be detri-
mental to the patient's well-being and have an adverse effect on
the progress of the disease and response to treatment. Perhaps
more importantly, people who, rightly or wrongly, believe that
they have a cancer become anxious and emotionally disturbed
even if they were not before. This is a natural and understandable reaction to what is often regarded as a death sentence at
worst, or a very serious illness requiring radical or prolonged
treatment and possibly disfigurement at best.

Such emotional distress will often cause patients to seek

alternative or fringe medicine therapists or faith healers or to fall prey to unqualified quacks, especially if they have been told that traditional medicine has nothing to offer.

These natural reactions should be anticipated by every doctor who cares for cancer patients. Support for the emotional needs of the patient and the patient's family should be readily available and considered in all situations. Sometimes this can be given effectively by the responsible clinicians with the cooperation and help of the family doctor and members of the nursing staff and other qualified helpers such as social workers, psychologists or members of the clergy or other spiritual advisors. Sometimes the help of an understanding psychiatrist experienced in this field is mandatory; certainly it is valuable for a cancer treatment team to have the services of an interested and experienced psychiatrist and/or clinical psychologist and a social worker.

Some psychiatrists and paramedical workers have claimed that some patients who have learned techniques of relaxation and meditation or hypnotherapy have shown not only emotional and physical benefit but even regression of the size of the cancer. In some traditions, acupuncture has given similar benefit. In some patients such benefits may be very real but they are difficult to evaluate, as cases of spontaneous cancer regression in response to no particular therapy have been reported in the medical literature. However, an experienced psychiatrist, clinical psychologist or social worker can help the cancer patient and members of his or her family adjust to the new situation and its associated emotional, social and other problems. A social worker can advise on agency support that may be available. For many people, especially those with advanced or incurable cancer, an experienced member of the clergy or other spiritual advisor can be invaluable.

Palliative care specialists

In recent years, doctors, nurses and paramedical workers have developed a new specialty in palliative care. These specialists have now become most valuable members of cancer treatment teams. Invariably understanding but also knowledgable in their patient care, they specialise in the relief of pain and other symptoms and helping both patients and their families and friends to adjust to different circumstances and different needs – especially where there is no prospect of a cure of the cancer.

Follow-up care

No matter what treatment is used in cancer management, it is important for patients to have regular medical follow-up examination. The purpose of this care is to detect and treat at an early stage any recurring problem, but it also gives patients confidence that any new problem will be detected and treated early. It is also important for doctors to keep accurate and continuing records of the long-term success or otherwise of treatment given so that improved treatments can be recorded and further developed.

For many cancers, if, after treatment for a period of two years there is no evidence of cancer, it is likely that the cancer has been cured. Indeed, for most cancers, a period of five years free of cancer indicates that cure is almost certain. Two of the more common cancers, however, require a longer period of regular follow-up, as evidence of disease can show up years later. These are melanoma and breast cancer. It seems that for these two cancers in particular the body's natural immune defences can keep the cancer under control for many years until something causes it to recur years later. These recurrent or residual cancers are often slowly growing and are often curable, provided they have been detected while still small and localised, hence the special need for continued follow-up of these patients.

Non-traditional and fringe medicine

There are almost limitless numbers of 'cancer cures' promoted by a variety of people ranging from well-intentioned non-traditional or fringe medicine practitioners on the one hand to misguided quacks and unscrupulous charlatans on the other. These 'cures' range from large doses of vitamins (especially vitamin C, vitamin E and other anti-oxidants) to preparations of herbs, a variety of plant extracts (one of the most publicised being an extract of apricot kernels, laetrile), diets (especially low-protein diets), to meditation, acupuncture, hypnotherapy and faith healing. At the other extreme are sleight-of-hand manoeuvres in which practitioners pretend to extract cancers painlessly.

Some of these non-traditional and fringe remedies are undoubtedly based on incidental observations and may have value unrecognised by the medical profession, as perhaps may some herbal mixtures, anti-oxidants or vitamin C therapy or diet therapy. Others, however, may be based on an incidental observation of a cancer patient who happened to undergo a spontaneous remission rather than on scientific knowledge.

Most such unconventional 'cures' have been investigated and found to be lacking by any measurable scientific analysis, but people who find themselves unable to face the reality of an incurable condition or radical surgery will often search for a more acceptable alternative. This is understandable and must be appreciated by cancer treatment teams, who must be prepared to spend time in advising and helping cancer patients in their mental and emotional as well as physical distress. At the same time, medical practitioners should not close their minds to the possibility that one day an idea might be proposed or an observation made by a non-traditional practitioner that could be of unquestionable value in cancer treatment. The medical profession and research scientists are aware of these possibilities, and most proposed new cancer 'cures' undergo some form of examination by appropriate authorities.

For some patients, alternative or unorthodox therapy can be very comforting and supportive, even though specific cancer healing properties are not known or not understood. Provided such therapy is helping the patient, is not harmful either physically or financially, and does not conflict with necessary treatment, it should be supported by the cancer treatment team.

The question of legalising voluntary euthanasia

This question has been the subject of much serious and passionate debate. It is not appropriate to attempt in this book to resolve the many conflicts raised.

In Australia people who promote euthanasia do so with the objective of allowing those who are suffering from prolonged and continuous pain and distress to end their lives with dignity with the help of three independent qualified doctors who agree that there is no reasonable alternative.

On the other hand, many people oppose euthanasia. Some oppose it on the basis of strongly held religious convictions, but others express reservations for one or more of the following reasons:

High standards of palliative care are becoming more freely available. Such care often restores a valuable period of life with good quality to people previously considered to be in a hopeless situation.

To give sufficient quantities of morphine or other pain relieving drugs is legal and does not require a change in

Cancer explained

legislation, even though it is appreciated that sooner or later the patient will succumb to the dose given.

People have the right to refuse artificial means of keeping alive their close family members or themselves if they are in an otherwise hopeless situation. Doctors are likewise discouraged from giving blood transfusions or other treatments to patients to prolong a hopeless condition.

Some people who have a depressive illness also develop another disease like cancer and may use the diagnosis of cancer to request help in suicide. Not all patients, even with advanced cancer, are prepared to acknowledge the benefits of pain relieving drugs or other good palliative care when they wish to end their lives for their own reasons.

Many doctors, nurses and other health professionals are unhappy that the highest ideals of their professions could become compromised if the role of 'takers of human life' were delegated to them. They would see their role as being quite different, and would prefer to be seen as people that patients can trust to preserve their lives with as little pain or distress as is possible.

Perhaps the greatest worry of all to most medical practitioners is that no matter where a line is drawn, there will always be exceptions that at first appear reasonable. Gradually the laws would be compromised, leading to abuse of the well informed, voluntary nature and other strict conditions of the system.

76

Some common cancers

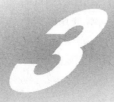

Skin cancers

Cancer of the skin is the cancer most commonly affecting people of European descent. It is especially common in fair-skinned people who live in sunny climates. Australians have the world's highest incidence of skin cancer, followed by the white populations of the southern regions of the USA.

There are three common types of skin cancer – basal cell carcinoma (BCC), which is by far the most common and, fortunately, the least dangerous; squamous cell carcinoma (SCC), which is the next most common; and melanoma, which is the least common of the three but the most dangerous.

BASAL CELL CARCINOMA

A basal cell carcinoma (BCC) is usually first noticed as a small, crusty patch or nodule or ulcer. These cancers occur most commonly in skin which has been constantly exposed to sunshine over many years. Hence they are not common before the age of 40 years and become more common with increasing age. More than 70% of these cancers occur on the face, as the skin of the face is most constantly exposed to the sun. The next most common sites are the neck, the backs of the hands or forearms, the lower legs, chest and back.

BCCs are not painful and are usually slow growing; patients may have noticed them for months or even years before they seek medical attention. If neglected, they usually develop as slowly enlarging ulcers (sometimes called 'rodent' ulcers because they may look like skin that has been gnawed by a rodent). Although, fortunately, they almost never spread to lymph nodes or other distant tissues, they do tend to erode locally into tissues around them. If neglected for a long time they may become incurable or even fatal by causing destruction to such tissues as underlying cartilage of the nose or ear, underlying bone of the skull, or large blood vessels in the neck. They can sometimes invade the orbit and paranasal sinuses and may even erode into the brain.

Treatment

BCCs can be easily and effectively cured in their early stages by simple surgical excision, usually under local anaesthesia. The specimen of tissue excised is examined by a pathologist to confirm that it was a BCC and that it was completely excised with an adequate margin of normal tissue. Radiotherapy is also an effective method of treating many BCCs, but preferably after a small biopsy has been taken to confirm the diagnosis. Radio-therapy has the advantage of avoiding surgical operation and of being a painless procedure; it has the disadvantage of requiring expensive specialised equipment and personnel and several treat-ment attendances, and leaves some permanent damage to a small patch of skin. Another disadvantage is that if no tissue is removed, there may be some doubt about the exact diagnosis of the lesion and whether it was completely eradicated. However, for many small lesions, especially in elderly patients, it may be the most appropriate form of treatment.

Sometimes small BCCs are removed by dermatologists (skin specialists) using cauterisation or a small curette (a scraping instrument). These techniques should be left to experienced experts, as a mistake in diagnosis or incomplete removal can lead to a greater problem.

BCCs that recur after previous failed attempts at treatment or those occurring close to vital structures such as a tear duct or an eyelid present special problems and require expert attention.

Large BCCs invading bone or other tissues may require extensive surgical procedures including reconstructive surgery. Occasionally they may even be quite incurable and are possibly best treated by palliative radiotherapy. (Palliative treatment is treatment which will give a patient relief by reducing the tumour or lessening its symptoms without being likely to cure it).

Although such advanced lesions are not common, they are disastrous when they do occur and can easily be prevented by correct treatment in their early stages. Hence the importance of people with small lesions seeking medical help early when BCCs are easily and completely curable.

SQUAMOUS CELL CARCINOMA

Squamous cell carcinomas (SCCs) are also most common on the skin of the face, especially the lower part of the face and lower lip, but may also occur commonly on the neck, the backs of the hands or forearms or skin of other frequently exposed areas such as the legs, back or chest.

They often develop in skin lesions called hyperkeratoses, which are small crusty or flaky thickened areas of skin resulting from previous longstanding sun damage.

An SCC is usually first noticed as a small painless lump growing on the skin's surface or as an ulcer in the skin. SCCs usually grow more rapidly than BCCs and after a time tend to spread to nearby draining lymph nodes. Later, they may even spread further to more distant lymph nodes or even to other distant tissues or organs such as the lung. They also grow locally and are likely to invade surrounding tissues which may ulcerate, bleed and become painful.

Fortunately, however, most SCCs of skin have not spread when they are first diagnosed, and treatment of draining lymph nodes is usually not required. However, draining lymph nodes must be kept under close observation and in case of enlargement should be treated without delay – usually by surgical excision.

Treatment

As for all cancers, the earlier these lesions are diagnosed and treated, the less radical treatment they need and the greater the likelihood of cure.

For any lesion suspected of being an SCC, it is important to obtain a tissue diagnosis – that is, for a biopsy to be taken. In the case of a small lesion, this may be best achieved by surgical excision of the whole lesion (an excision biopsy). For a large lesion it is usually more appropriate for a small piece of tissue to be taken from its edge for biopsy and microscopic examination (an incision biopsy). A frozen section examination of a biopsy specimen, as described in Section 2, may be appropriate to allow complete treatment to be carried out without delay.

Once the diagnosis of an SCC is established, treatment is usually by surgical excision or sometimes by radiotherapy. Surgical excision is usually the most effective and most appropriate treatment. The lesion is widely excised and examined microscopically to confirm that a margin of normal tissue surrounding the cancer has also been excised to ensure that removal of all the primary cancer has been achieved. If draining lymph nodes are enlarged, without evidence that this is due to infection, the lymph nodes should also be removed, in one block of tissue. Depending on the site and how much tissue has to be excised, a plastic surgical procedure such as a skin graft may be needed to repair the tissue and close the wound.

As in the case of BCCs, radiotherapy may be used to treat some SCCs of skin, especially in elderly patients, in patients for whom an operation might be risky or occasionally as palliative treatment when cure by surgery is not possible.

Occasionally, when an SCC of skin is very advanced, or invading vital organs or other tissues, or has become incurable because of secondary spread, it may be appropriate to use anti-cancer drugs to reduce the extent and size of the cancer and to relieve symptoms. People occasionally are seen with large SCCs of skin which appear incurable by radiotherapy or surgery (or only curable by mutilating surgery such as amputation of a limb). These can sometimes be reduced in size and extent by chemo-therapy first, especially when given regionally by intra-arterial infusion (as described in Section 2). After chemotherapy, the tumours are often so reduced in size, extent and viability that they have been converted into small tumours which can then be cured by radiotherapy and/or local surgical excision.

MELANOMA

Melanoma is the most dangerous form of skin cancer. A mela-noma is a malignant growth of pigment-forming cells in skin or in an eye. Occasionally they may occur in mucous membranes such as the lining of the mouth or anus.

Although melanoma is a highly malignant tumour, present-day management methods have greatly improved the outlook. Considered almost universally fatal 40 or 50 years ago, mela-noma can now be cured in more than 80% of cases.

The cause of melanoma is not known, although it is most common in fair-skinned people living in sunny tropical or subtropical climates. As opposed to BCCs and SCCs, however, melanoma does not commonly occur on areas of the body most constantly exposed to sunshine. The most common sites are on the backs of men or on the thighs of women, as opposed to the face, which is the most common site of other cancers caused by sunshine. However, in common with other skin cancers, the world's highest incidence of melanoma is in the white population of Australia, especially those living closest to the equator and nearest to the seaside. The white population of the sunny southern parts of the USA also has a high incidence of melanoma. People of dark-skinned races do occasionally develop a melanoma, but in these people it is more common to be at sites of less pigmentation such as the sole of the foot, under fingernails or toenails or in the mucosa lining the mouth or anus.

Melanoma rarely affects children before puberty, but after puberty it can affect people of any age including teenagers and young adults as well as middle-aged and older people. Although it affects males and females almost equally, the outlook for females is rather better than that for males.

The danger of melanoma lies in the fact that it tends to spread early to draining lymph nodes and to distant organs such as the liver, lungs, bowel wall and brain. The outlook has improved recently mainly because people in general, and doctors in particular, are becoming more aware of the early indications of melanoma and of the need to commence treatment as early as possible. Most melanomas develop in pre-existing moles in the skin, but others develop in areas of skin without any pre-existing mole. Occasionally a melanoma will develop without pigment. This is known as an amelanotic melanoma and can be diagnosed only by microscopic examination. Amelanotic melanomas behave in a way similar to pigmented melanomas and require similar treatment.

Symptoms and signs

Any evidence of increasing pigmentation in a spot in the skin, especially an increase in size or pigmentation of a mole, must be regarded with suspicion. Other early features may be itching or crusting of a mole. Bleeding and ulceration are usually later features. Any of these features occurring either in a pre-existing mole or in a newly pigmented spot require immediate attention, and if there is any doubt, a biopsy should be taken. This is often best done by a surgeon who has expert frozen section facilities available and is prepared to go ahead with appropriate surgical treatment if the biopsy proves positive.

Treatment

Surgical excision of early lesions offers the best hope of cure. The melanoma must be excised with a wide margin of normal surrounding tissue as its cells are sometimes present in tissues or even in lymphatic vessels surrounding the tumour. If there is evidence of draining lymph node involvement, then these lymph nodes should also be excised in one block of tissue. The likelihood of spread of melanoma is directly related to the thickness of the tumour, so that in the case of thick lesions, excision of lymph nodes may be considered even though they are not found to be enlarged. In specialised melanoma units, special X-ray-like tests have been used to try to detect whether nearby draining lymph nodes appear to be normal or whether they have defects that may indicate the presence of melanoma cells. These tests (lymph node scintigraphy) are *not* proving helpful in deciding whether or not lymph nodes contain metastatic melanoma, but they do indicate which lymph nodes are most likely to be involved and therefore which nodes, if any, should be considered for excision and examination.

Melanomas are not particularly sensitive to radiotherapy, although radiotherapy may be helpful in some situations such as for a secondary melanoma in the brain. Chemotherapy has in general been disappointing in treating melanoma. Occasional beneficial responses have been observed, but they are all too infrequent. When advanced melanoma appears to be confined to one limb, treatment by more concentrated regional chemotherapy via a special technique – into the blood supply of that limb only – often achieves worthwhile improvement, with tumour regression. This technique is called 'closed circuit perfusion'. A newer, more easily used technique is 'closed circuit infusion'. This treatment is more effective if heat is used with the chemotherapy and appears to be even more effective if a new immunotherapy agent TNF (tumour necrosis factor) is used with chemotherapy.

Immunotherapy is also sometimes used in treatment of advanced or widespread melanoma. Although some improvements have been observed with general (systemic) immunotherapy, most results have been inconsistent, and early hopes of a reliable new cure have not yet been fulfilled.

Work with chemotherapy and immunotherapy is continuing in melanoma clinics in the hope of improving treatment techniques so that more reliable treatment methods may be available for advanced melanoma in the future.

Lung cancer

Cancer of the lung has increased from being an uncommon disease at the turn of the century to one which in males now causes more deaths than any other cancer. This rapid increase in incidence is directly related to the widespread habit of cigarette smoking – the disease being eight to 10 times more common in smokers than in non-smokers. With greater numbers of females smoking in recent years, the incidence of lung cancer in women is now approaching that of men.

Although tobacco smoking is by far the most significant cause, a number of other factors may also play a part in some cases, including industrial and automobile pollutant gases. Workers in certain industries including the chromium, arsenic and asbestos industries also have an increased incidence, especially if they are also smokers.

Symptoms and signs

During its early stages, lung cancer causes few problems, so that it is usually not diagnosed until it is quite advanced and often incurable. Perhaps this is partly because of the nature of the sufferer who, being a smoker, is used to having a chronic cough and does not become aware of a change in the cough until the disease is advanced. A cough is the most common single symptom of lung cancer, but other features are shortness of breath, coughing up blood or blood-stained sputum, chest pain and attacks of chest infection or pneumonia which do not settle down completely with treatment.

The first evidence of lung cancer can also be provided by secondary cancers in lymph nodes, bone, brain or elsewhere. Sometimes lung cancers produce hormones or other substances which may affect the sufferer as a whole and result in changes in other parts of the body such as swelling of the breasts, changes in bones, or fingernails, or loss of nerve function, which may cause numbness or tingling sensations.

Investigations

Chest X-rays sometimes show a lung cancer that has not been causing symptoms, but by the time symptoms are present, X-rays will show the cancer in most cases.

CT scans may also show more clearly the position and the size of a lung cancer.

Bronchoscopy (examination of the air passages with a bronchoscope) will often allow the doctor to see a lung cancer. A biopsy of the suspected cancer may be taken and examined under a microscope to confirm that cancer is present, to find out what sort of lung cancer it is, and therefore how best to treat it.

Sometimes a cancer cannot be seen through a bronchoscope but can be detected in sputum that has been sucked out or coughed up and examined under a microscope. This test is called cytology. It will often show cancer cells if a cancer is present. If a lump is seen on X-ray, sometimes it is possible to suck out cells for cytology from the lump through a needle inserted through the chest wall (see Section 2).

Treatment

Most people with lung cancer do not notice symptoms early and do not seek treatment until the disease has spread from the lung into surrounding structures, lymph nodes or other parts of the body. At this stage it may be incurable. For those who do seek treatment early and are diagnosed when their cancers are small and possibly curable, the best results are achieved by an operation to remove all or part of a lung. However, relatively few can be cured in the long term because they are not diagnosed early enough.

Radiotherapy is sometimes used when surgery is unsuitable, but cure by radiotherapy alone is uncommon. Results of chemotherapy and immunotherapy for lung cancer have been disappointing as a whole, although newer anti-cancer drugs used by experts in certain combinations and in certain treatment programs can achieve worthwhile improvement for some types of lung cancer. The improvement may last for several months or even a year or two. Combinations of newer chemotherapy schedules used with radiotherapy and/or surgery may have more to offer in the future. Such combinations of drugs with other treatments are being investigated in a number of leading cancer treatment centres throughout the world.

MESOTHELIOMA

Mesothelioma is a rare form of cancer that is well known to some industrial workers: when it does occur it is usually in people who have been exposed to asbestos in their work. Asbestos workers who are also smokers are particularly at risk. Industrial laws that protect asbestos workers from this hazard have kept this as an uncommon cancer.

Mesothelioma is not truly a cancer of the lung but is a cancer of the tissues surrounding and lining the lungs (the pleura). It may rarely occur in other lining tissues such as the lining of the abdominal cavity (the peritoneum). Mesothelioma patients may seek treatment for a cough, chest infection, difficulty with breathing or chest pain. A tumour lump may be felt or seen on an X-ray or CT scan.

Mesothelioma is difficult to treat, as it is usually too widespread and advanced to treat by surgery and does not usually respond well to either radiotherapy or chemotherapy. The best treatment is often simply to give the patient best relief from symptoms while the tumour progresses slowly.

SECONDARY CANCER IN THE LUNG

The lungs are among the organs most commonly the site of secondary growths from cancers growing in other parts of the body. Cancers from almost any primary site are likely to spread through the bloodstream to the lungs, especially from cancers of the breast, kidney, bone, ovary or from melanoma of skin. These usually show as a number of rounded opacities (white spots) on chest X-rays, although sometimes a secondary (especially from the kidney), may be single, showing as just one round white spot on an X-ray. Treatment depends on the type of cancer that has spread to the lung, but in general anti-cancer drugs are more likely to be helpful than any other anti-cancer treatment. However, as cure is unlikely, treatment with risk of troublesome side-effects may or may not be considered worthwhile. Occasionally there may be hope for a cure when there is only one secondary seen in the lung X-ray (especially if it has come from a cancer of kidney or a sarcoma of bone or soft tissue which has been successfully removed), and it may be possible for a surgeon to remove that part of the lung affected.

Sometimes primary or secondary cancer in the lung will cause fluid to collect around the lung in the pleural cavity. This is known as a pleural effusion. Pleural effusion causes shortness of breath and difficulty with breathing as a result of pressure on the lung. Sometimes patients will get good relief from the removal of this fluid with a needle and syringe. Injection of an anti-cancer drug into the pleural cavity after the removal of the fluid may slow the rate at which fluid collects in the cavity.

Breast cancer

Breast cancer is becoming more common in westernised societies, and apart from skin cancer, is now the most common cancer affecting women in the USA and Australia. About one in 11 American women will develop breast cancer during her lifetime. Although occasionally seen in women in their twenties, breast cancer is not common until after the age of 40 years and becomes more common with increasing age. The average age for women with breast cancer is about 60 years.

Although the cause of breast cancer is not known, there are a number of associated factors. The one most recognised significant factor is probably the age of a woman when she has her first baby. Having a baby at an early age seems to give some protection: breast cancer is least common in women who had their first babies as teenagers and significantly more common in women who did not have their first baby until after the age of 30 or 35 years. Women who have not had children are at greater risk from breast cancer.

The age of onset of menstruation and the age at menopause are also significant. Early menstruation and late menopause are both associated with an increased risk of breast cancer. It seems that the longer the woman's reproductive life cycle, the greater the risk of breast cancer.

There may also be some protection in breastfeeding, although the evidence for this is less clear. Women who live in undeveloped countries tend to breastfeed their babies for many months and have a low risk of breast cancer. However, these women also usually have had their first baby at a young age and have usually had a very different diet from women of Western countries.

There is an association between breast cancer and a diet high in animal fat, being overweight and tobacco smoking, although these associations are not as obvious as tobacco smoking and lung cancer.

Breast injury has sometimes been suspected, but it is really not known whether this may cause a breast cancer. Although some women first notice a lump which is found to be breast cancer after injury, it is likely that in most cases the injury simply drew attention to a cancer lump which was already present. Injuries may, of course, cause other types of lumps in the breast which are not cancer.

Hormone replacement therapy (HRT) has been incriminated as increasing the risk of breast cancer. However, unless the woman had previously been treated for breast cancer or has some special risk factor (such as a strong family history of breast cancer) the risk of small doses of hormones is very small. HRT is therefore not given to every woman who reaches the menopause, but for those having severe menopausal or post-menopausal problems the possible very small risk may well be justified provided the woman is kept under regular observation. Meanwhile, studies continue to try to find something equally effective, but without risk, to relieve these symptoms. One study is investigating the hormones that occur naturally in soy beans and other plant foods, the phytoestrogens.

Cancer in the male breast occasionally occurs but it is uncommon. Fewer than 1% of all breast cancers are in males, but when they do occur in males they show up and behave in a similar way to cancer in female breasts, although the outlook for breast cancer in males is usually worse than that for breast cancer in females.

Symptoms and signs

Breast cancer is usually first noticed when a woman finds a pain-less lump in the breast. The most common location is in the upper outer part of the breast, and the lump is often first felt in the bath when fingers are soapy and lumps are more obvious.

Of course, all breast lumps are not cancer. By far the majority of breast lumps are not cancer. However, when a woman first notices a lump in a breast, she should have it examined by a doctor. If necessary the woman should be sent for further inves-tigation or for a specialist opinion.

Other features of breast cancer may be a change in the posi-tion or shape of a nipple (called retraction or inversion); redness, puckering or ulceration of skin over the breast–especially if over a lump; discharge of blood from a nipple or discharge of other fluid from a nipple not associated with a pregnancy or lactation; redness of a nipple; or a change in size of one breast. Occasionally the first indication of breast cancer is a red inflamed breast very like breast infection (acute mastitis). If an 'acute mastitis' develops for no apparent reason or does not settle down with appropriate treatment (including antibiotics), the possibility of an underlying cancer must be considered.

Sometimes breast cancer may first be discovered after finding a lump in the armpit (axilla) or a tumour lump (secondary) in another organ such as in lungs (seen in a chest X-ray), liver or bone.

The doctor usually looks for a breast lump with special features of being hard, irregular in outline and possibly firmly attached to skin, muscle or other tissue. The doctor will examine lymph nodes in the armpit or elsewhere for evidence of enlargement and will also examine the chest and abdomen for possible evidence of lumps or spread into other organs such as lungs, liver, ovaries, etc.

Investigations

Screening tests for breast cancer are discussed in Section 2. A number of investigations are available for detecting breast cancer. Breast X-rays (mammograms) may show the type of lump and the general condition of the breast. Ultrasound and CT scans may also be helpful, although as a rule they give little further information.

The most important investigation is a biopsy. In many cases a needle biopsy may be carried out on an outpatient basis. Sometimes it is better for a surgeon to take a larger biopsy in an operating theatre: this is the most reliable method of diagnosis. If a surgical biopsy is carried out with a frozen section pathology technique (described in Section 2), the surgeon can usually go ahead with any necessary surgical operation without further delay.

If, after a doctor's examination, a breast lump is thought to be cancer, and especially if it is an advanced cancer, other general investigations may be arranged. These may include chest X-rays, liver scans and bone scans, or CT scans, which may provide evidence of possible spread to lungs, liver or bone. The involvement of any of these organs should be known before any major surgery is carried out on the breast. If other organs are affected, some form of treatment other than removal of the breast may be more appropriate.

Treatment

Treatment of breast cancer will depend on whether the cancer was detected early and is likely to be cured by surgery or other local treatment, or whether it is so advanced that cure by treatment of the breast alone is not possible.

Prevention

There is no known practical way of preventing the development of breast cancer apart from possibly a change in traditional diets and lifestyle of girls and young women from high-risk communities. However, studies are presently being conducted on the use of the anti-oestrogen hormone compound tamoxifen, given in small doses over a prolonged period of years, to prevent breast cancer developing in women at special risk. Women at special risk are those with a very high incidence of breast cancer in their immediate family or those who have already had cancer in one breast. Results of these trials and the risks of this treatment are not yet fully known.

Further studies at the time of writing are based on the fact that women in Asian countries have a lower incidence of breast cancer and premenstrual syndrome than women in Western societies. Asian women have a diet high in soy beans and other foods that contain the natural hormone substances known as the phytoestrogens. The present studies are designed to determine whether the phytoestrogens from these dietary products reduce the risk of breast diseases including cancer.

EARLY BREAST CANCER
Surgery and/or radiotherapy

No cancer treatment is more controversial than the treatment of early breast cancer.

For many years, surgeons have believed that if a cancer is small and is only in the breast or in the breast and possibly the small lymph nodes in the armpit, then the best chance of cure was by total removal of the breast and all draining lymph nodes in the armpit. This operation, known as radical mastectomy, has been used for many years and has cured many women of breast cancer.

More recently, studies seem to show that results of treatment are just as good if only the breast is removed and lymph nodes are treated by radiotherapy.

Some other studies suggest that results may be equally good if only that part of the breast containing the lump is removed and the remainder of the breast and lymph nodes are treated by radiotherapy.

The exact truth in all of these different claims and studies is hard to find, as it is difficult to compare results from one hospital with those of another, or even to compare different groups of patients in the one hospital or group of hospitals. The age of patients, the size and type and position of the cancers, the degree of involvement of lymph nodes, the skill of surgeons or radiotherapists, and the number of years of follow-up studies all present so many variables that exact comparisons cannot be made.

It is probably true that, although logic suggests that radical mastectomy should be most likely to result in a cure, if there is any difference in cure rates compared with other forms of treatment it must be very small; therefore the patient's wishes should be taken into consideration. If the patient would prefer to have the breast with a cancer in it totally removed, then this treatment should be offered. On the other hand, where a patient has a very strong wish not to lose all of her breast, and the surgeon cannot assure her that radical removal of the breast is more likely to cure her, a less radical operation with radiotherapy would seem more appropriate.

Adjuvant chemotherapy

Whatever the initial form of treatment, it is now appreciated that in a number of women with breast cancer apparently confined to the breast and nearby lymph nodes, there will also be early but undetectable spread of some cancer cells to other parts of the body such as the lungs, liver, bones or elsewhere. If chemotherapy is given at this stage, the very small clumps of scattered cancer cells, if present, are more likely to be destroyed than if they are allowed to get bigger before any effective treatment is given. In women who have had an early breast cancer removed and cancer has also been found in the lymph nodes in the armpit, in spite of the fact that there is no proof that the cancer has spread any further, there is a real chance that it has. For this reason, a program of chemotherapy is usually given after the operation. This is known as adjuvant chemotherapy, the chemotherapy being an adjunct or assistant to the surgery. Women given adjuvant chemotherapy are less likely to develop secondary cancer and are therefore more likely to be cured. As indicated in Section 2, the chemotherapy must be given skilfully and the effects watched closely, as side-effects are common. Adjuvant chemotherapy is more appropriate for younger women, who appear to benefit more and also tolerate better the effects of chemotherapy than do older women. Tamoxifen therapy is usually more appropriate for older women.

ADVANCED BREAST CANCER

Women with advanced breast cancer such as cancer fungating (ulcerating) through the skin of the breast or cancer with secondary spread to other tissues or organs are unlikely to be cured by local surgery alone. Sometimes chemotherapy or radiotherapy or both may be given first to reduce the tumour size, and sometimes this may be followed by surgical removal of the breast to prevent further local growth or fungation. Treatment of advanced cancer in the breast by chemotherapy (and possibly intra-arterial chemotherapy) followed by radiotherapy and then mastectomy (see Section 2) has resulted in cure in some cases that would previously have been regarded as incurable due to advanced cancers in the breast involving surrounding tissues like skin and muscle. However, for such advanced local cancers, especially with distant secondary cancers in other tissues, the best palliation may often be achieved by some form of hormonal treatment (some breast cancers being sensitive to hormones) or by chemotherapy alone. (Hormone treatment is discussed in Section 2.) In some cases secondary cancers may respond well to radiotherapy. This is especially appropriate for isolated, painful secondary cancers in bone.

Treatment of complications may also be required to give the patient relief from distressing symptoms such as fluid in the chest (pleural cavity) or treatment of pain (as discussed in Section 2); blood transfusions may be given to relieve symptoms of anaemia.

There are now two new research approaches under study in breast cancer treatment. The first, for advanced breast cancer, is bone marrow transplantation after intense chemotherapy. Some success has been reported from this approach. The other new approach is gene therapy, in which abnormal genetic material in cancer cells is replaced with non-malignant genetic material.

Although at the time of writing techniques are still being developed to make this approach clinically effective, this therapy is causing a great deal of research interest.

Breast prostheses and breast reconstruction

After loss of a breast, many women feel quite depressed, even humiliated, and require sympathetic help and understanding.

Breast prosthetic padding has improved, and types are now available that allow normal activity, even swimming, without detection. In other cases, surgery by a surgeon who specialises in plastic or reconstructive surgery may be considered. These procedures are usually not advised until at least a couple of years after mastectomy, in order to be as sure as possible that recurrence of the cancer is unlikely. On the other hand, some surgeons are now offering reconstructive surgery to replace the breast immediately after its removal. Such procedures offer considerable emotional support to some women, although the long-term results of early reconstruction are as yet uncertain.

Emotional support and the understanding of family and friends are essential for most women who have had breast cancer, especially if they have had a mastectomy. As breast cancer is one of the most common cancers in Western societies, many cities will have a **mastectomy club** that women are welcome to join. Company and advice from fellow club members can be of great help in meeting both the physical and emotional needs of such women.

Cancers of the digestive system

CANCER OF THE OESOPHAGUS

The oesophagus is the hollow food passage that passes through the chest joining the mouth and pharynx (in the neck) to the stomach (in the abdomen). Cancer of the oesophagus is a common disease in Japan, China and other Asian and some African countries as well as Russia and Scandinavia, but is less common in Britain, America, Canada, Australia, New Zealand and the white population of South Africa. The reason for this difference in incidence is not fully understood. It has often been suggested that diet plays a part. In some parts of China with a very high incidence of cancer of the oesophagus, a fungus that grows on poorly stored food may be at least partly responsible. Cancer of the oesophagus is more common in men than in women and like cancers in the mouth and throat, it is more common in smokers and heavy drinkers of alcohol than in non-smokers and non-drinkers.

Symptoms and signs

Unfortunately, cancer of the oesophagus is usually well established before it is diagnosed. The most common symptom is difficulty with swallowing. First there is difficulty in swallowing solid foods, which seem to get caught in the throat or chest. Later, there is difficulty in swallowing liquids. A person with cancer of the oesophagus thus soon loses weight and may become quite wasted and even dehydrated.

Investigations

Barium swallow or barium meal X-rays (see Section 2) will usually show an obstruction to swallowing in the oesophagus and an irregular narrowing at the site of the cancer.

Oesophagoscopy is carried out. Through the oesophagoscope the doctor can usually see an irregular or ulcerated tumour. A biopsy will be taken to establish the diagnosis under the microscope.

Unfortunately, cancers of the oesophagus have usually spread up and down the mucous membrane (lining) of the oesophagus and into lymph nodes and other structures in the chest before the patient notices many symptoms. Thus these cancers are very often not curable when first seen by the doctor.

Treatment

The best hope of cure is by surgery. The oesophagus is removed and either the stomach or a section of bowel is used to make a new oesophagus for the passage of food.

Radiotherapy is also used to treat this cancer. Although it usually makes the cancer smaller for a period and relieves symptoms temporarily, it does not often cure it.

Radiotherapy and surgery are sometimes used together, but results are still not good.

Chemotherapy has also been disappointing in treating this cancer. Attempts some years ago to get better results by using chemotherapy first to reduce the cancer and then surgery to remove the remaining cancer did not improve the results. However, recent efforts to get better results by such combined treatment with different drugs and treatment programs now being investigated may offer better hope for the future.

Sometimes it is not possible to attempt to remove the cancer, and the most helpful treatment is for the surgeon to pass a plastic tube through the oesophagus into the stomach to allow the patient to swallow food. Otherwise, some alternative food passage (such as a transplanted section of bowel) or another method of feeding may be required.

CANCER OF THE STOMACH

Cancer of the stomach has in the past been one of the more serious and more common cancers, but over recent years, it has become less common and continues to become less common.

Stomach cancer is uncommon before the age of 40 years but thereafter increases in incidence with age, reaching a peak between the ages of 60 and 65 years. Males are affected about two or three times more commonly than females.

Cancer of the stomach has a distinct racial or geographic association. It is about seven times more common in Japan and Korea and three or four times more common in eastern Europe than it is in the USA. Epidemiological studies suggest that it has a direct relationship to diet. People who have a diet high in animal fats and low in fresh fruit and vegetables are at greater risk of stomach cancer. It may also be related to a high intake of chemical food preservatives and food subject to other methods of preservation and preparation. The high intake of smoked fish in Japan has been incriminated; there is also a high incidence of this cancer among people of northern Iceland, who eat large amounts of crude smoked salmon as opposed to a lower incidence in the people of southern Iceland who have a different diet. In Korea, the custom of eating a great deal of red pepper and possibly other spices in food is thought to be significant.

It has been suggested that the decreasing incidence of stomach cancer in modern industrialised societies is the result of the greater availability of fresh fruit and vegetables due to modern quick transport and the use of refrigeration to store food rather than subjecting it to chemical preservatives and additives.

Other conditions that result in a higher risk of stomach cancer are pernicious anaemia (people with pernicious anaemia have about six times the normal risk of developing a stomach cancer), chronic gastritis, polyps in the stomach and possibly gastric ulcers. Smokers also have an increased risk compared to non-smokers.

Symptoms and signs

Like cancer of the oesophagus, cancer of the stomach is usually quite advanced before pain or other symptoms are noticed. The

earliest symptom is usually some vague indigestion that gradually gets worse and more persistent. Persistent indigestion occurring for the first time in someone over the age of 40 years must
always be considered with suspicion.

Sometimes an early feature is loss of appetite especially for
certain foods – a loss of appetite for meat is common. Other
symptoms may be a feeling of being full or even feeling 'blown
up' in the stomach after eating small amounts of food or
vomiting after food, particularly if vomiting becomes frequent or
regular. If a cancer has blocked the stomach, vomiting becomes
persistent. Pain is sometimes the first symptom, but when pain
is persistent, the cancer is often quite advanced.

Sometimes a patient has not been aware of any symptoms
but has found a lump in the upper abdomen. In others, symptoms of feeling weak and tired due to anaemia or recent unex-
plained weight loss may have caused the patient to seek medical
attention without noticing any particular indigestion or abdominal complaints. Occasionally the first evidence of trouble is
caused by the cancer spreading to other organs or tissues: an
enlarged liver, or jaundice, or pain in the back can be caused by
the cancer spreading to the pancreas or other tissues behind the
stomach (see Figure 1).

The doctor will look for a swelling or lump in the abdomen,
evidence of enlarged liver or lymph nodes (especially an enlarged
lymph node in the left side of the neck), evidence of spread into
the pelvis or an ovary (felt on vaginal or rectal examination), or
evidence of fluid in the abdominal cavity. There might also be
anaemia or weight loss.

Investigations

The doctor may test for blood in the faeces or test blood for
anaemia or other abnormalities.

Barium meal X-ray films and screening (see Section 2) may

show an ulcer (usually with raised, rounded edges), or a lump on the stomach wall looking something like a small cauliflower. The X-rays and screening may alternatively show a blocked stomach, a change in the stomach's shape or size (bigger or shrunken and smaller), or a more rigid and stiff-walled stomach. However, X-rays will not show all cancers in the stomach and other tests are also needed.

Gastroscopy (see Section 2) is a very useful investigation. Through a gastroscope a cancer can not only be seen as an ulcer with raised edges, a cauliflower-like mass or rigid abnormal distortion of the stomach wall, but a biopsy can also be taken to confirm the diagnosis and to determine the type of cancer. Present-day gastroscopy is now a common test and can be performed without stress to the patient; it is now usually performed before barium meal X-ray studies.

CT scans may be useful to determine the size and exact position of a cancer. It may show, for example, spread into the pancreas behind the stomach or spread into the liver. A liver isotope scan may also show evidence of spread into the liver.

Treatment

The only method for the cure of cancer of the stomach is by surgical operation in which either all of the stomach is removed (total gastrectomy); most of the stomach is removed (sub-total gastrectomy); or part of the stomach is removed (partial gastrectomy).

If a cancer has already spread beyond the stomach it may not be possible to cure the patient by surgery, but it may still be possible to give the patient relief of symptoms by a non-curative operation such as an operation to relieve any blockage of the stomach.

After total gastrectomy, the small intestine is joined to the oesophagus or, in the case of a sub-total or partial gastrectomy, the small intestine is joined to the small remaining part of the stomach to allow food to pass through normally. With no stomach present or only a small part of the stomach present, the patient can eat only small meals and therefore needs to eat frequently to avoid excessive weight loss. Without a stomach the patient may also develop anaemia, and will be given treatment to prevent this.

Results of surgery alone in treating stomach cancer have been disappointing in the past. In general, the smaller a cancer is at surgery the better the results. For this reason, gastroscopy and other diagnostic tests may be used to look for evidence of cancer as soon as a patient complains to a doctor of early symptoms, especially if the patient is a male over the age of 40 years. In some countries, and especially in Japan, screening tests are often carried out for people at risk even though they may not have any symptoms. When stomach cancers are found while they are small and in the early stages (as is now often the case in Japan), results of treatment by operation are good, with a high rate of cure. However, this is not often the case in Western societies, where stomach cancer is less common and is not often diagnosed until troublesome symptoms have developed, by which time the cancers are advanced and unlikely to be cured by surgery alone.

Anti-cancer drugs do not cure this cancer, but they may be useful in treating people whose cancers cannot be cured by operation. The drugs will often make the cancers smaller and may give the patients good relief, possibly for several months.

More recently, anti-cancer drugs have been given to some patients before the operation is carried out (*induction or neoadjuvant chemotherapy* – see Section 2). There is some evidence that if the cancers are made smaller by the drugs and then the operation (gastrectomy) is carried out, the results and the chances of cure will be better. The most effective way of giving the anti-cancer chemotherapy before operation may be by administering the drugs directly into the artery that supplies blood to the stomach. After a month or so of giving the drugs this way, the cancer is often smaller and the chances of curing the patient by operation may be better.

More studies of these techniques are needed, but there is some hope of getting better results with treatment of stomach cancer in the future by one or both of these two newer approaches. Firstly, by earlier diagnostic tests to detect cancers at an earlier and more curable stage and, secondly, by the use of initial chemotherapy followed by surgery for those people who seek treatment with well established but removable cancers.

CANCER OF THE LIVER

PRIMARY LIVER CANCER (HEPATOMA)

Cancer starting in liver cells (primary cancer) is uncommon in European races but is common in Africans, South-East Asians, Chinese and Japanese. It ranges as high as half of all cancers in African Bantu men. The reasons for this difference in incidence are not completely understood, although differences in diet and food storage are probably important. Longstanding liver infection with hepatitis B and hepatitis C and parasitic infestation, particularly by the liver fluke, are responsible for much of the increased incidence in the Orient. Certain fungi that commonly contaminate food in parts of Africa and Asia may also play a part, whereas food stored by refrigeration in westernised societies is almost invariably free from such contamination.

Primary liver cancer also sometimes develops in people with longstanding cirrhosis of the liver, whether the cirrhosis is the result of excessive alcohol consumption or other causes.

Symptoms and signs

The first evidence of primary liver cancer may be of general ill health (loss of appetite, weight loss, weakness and debility) or features of liver enlargement with pain in the upper abdomen, swelling, jaundice or fluid in the abdominal cavity (ascites).

Investigations

Investigations that may help include isotope liver scans, CT scans, ultrasound, sometimes arteriography, but especially liver biopsy (see Section 2). Blood tests for liver function, for anaemia and for blood chemical changes are often helpful. A special tumour marker test called alpha-feto-protein estimation is usually found to give an elevated reading in people with this cancer; it usually falls to normal levels if the cancer has been cured. Progressive alpha-feto-protein tests may give useful evidence of the effectiveness of treatment.

Treatment

Treatment of primary liver cancer is only successful if the disease is detected when it is confined to a part of the liver that can be removed by surgical operation. As the cancer has usually spread widely in the liver when first detected, cure is usually not possible.

SECONDARY LIVER CANCER

Although primary liver cancer is uncommon in people of European races, the liver is one of the most common sites of secondary cancer in all races including Europeans. Cancers of the digestive tract, especially the stomach, pancreas, colon and rectum, commonly spread via the bloodstream to the liver. Cancers of almost any other tissue may also spread to the liver, but breast cancer, lung cancer and melanoma are especially likely to do this.

Secondary cancers in the liver cause it to enlarge. It may become uncomfortable or even painful, jaundice often develops and fluid may accumulate in the abdominal cavity. A person with secondary liver cancer sooner or later notices loss of appetite, loss of weight and loss of energy. Breathlessness may also develop.

Investigations

The doctor will look for the features mentioned above and may arrange investigations to help establish the diagnosis. The most helpful investigations are usually the liver isotope scan, the CT scan, ultrasound and sometimes arteriography. A liver biopsy, either carried out with a special needle through the lower chest or abdominal wall under local anaesthesia or carried out at operation, may be required to be sure of the diagnosis, although very often it is obvious without carrying out this test.

If the site of a primary cancer that has spread to the liver is not known, investigations will also be carried out to discover where the secondary cancer in the liver originated.

Treatment

Secondary cancer in the liver is usually not a curable condition. The only hope of cure is where there are only one or two secondary cancers in a part of the liver that can be removed by an operation. This is not common. In most people the secondary cancers are spread throughout most parts of the liver.

Although there is no cure for most patients, some secondary cancers are sensitive to anti-cancer drugs. Secondary cancers in the liver that have come from primary cancer of the colon or rectum, stomach or breast are often sensitive to anti-cancer drugs.

Although the drugs do not totally cure the secondary cancers, they may make them smaller and sometimes give the patient good relief for some months.

The most simple method of giving such anti-cancer drugs is either by mouth or by injection into a vein, but a more effective method is by administering the drugs directly into the artery that supplies blood to the liver. This is called intra-arterial infusion chemotherapy (see Section 2).

Intra-arterial infusion chemotherapy can usually be given only in a hospital, with the patient returning for treatment at intervals as necessary. A few years ago a small pump was developed in America to continuously pump anti-cancer drugs into the artery supplying blood to the liver. This pump is implanted by a surgeon under the skin of the abdomen, where it stays without discomfort to the patient. It allows the patient having intra-arterial infusion chemotherapy to go home and lead a relatively normal life, returning for re-filling of the pump by simple injection into the pump once every week or every two weeks. The pump is expensive and suitable only for certain patients using certain drugs, but most patients with a pump live happily and comfortably for several months or even two or three years or more. For many of these patients, their time of survival has been increased with good quality of life. Other studies are being made to develop less expensive and more easily available methods of giving similar relief to greater numbers of patients using the principle of intra-arterial chemotherapy.

CANCER OF THE GALL BLADDER AND BILE DUCTS

These are uncommon cancers in Western countries, although quite common in some countries such as South India. Cancer of the gall bladder is usually associated with gallstones that have been present for many years. Hence it is more common in women of the older age group (as gallstones are more common in women). Cancer of the bile ducts, on the other hand, is slightly more common in men.

One reason for surgeons advising removal of gall bladders with gallstones, especially in young women, is that there is a risk that over the years a cancer may develop.

Early cancer may occasionally be found unexpectedly and incidentally on examination of the gall bladder after it has been removed for other reasons. In such cases, cure of the cancer may have been achieved simply by the removal of the gall bladder.

If not diagnosed early, cancer of the gall bladder may cause persistent pain in the upper right side of the abdomen, with evidence of inflammation of the gall bladder, or it may cause a swelling or lump felt in the upper abdomen under the ribs on the right side.

The first indication of cancer of the gall bladder, and more especially cancer of the bile ducts, may be jaundice due to the blockage of the flow of bile from the liver. The jaundice is often accompanied by a severe itch of the patient's skin.

Cancer of the gall bladder tends to spread into the liver as well as into nearby lymph nodes. Once this has happened it has become virtually incurable by surgery and does not respond well to radiotherapy. It also has a reputation for not responding well to chemotherapy, although good response to intra-arterial chemotherapy (see Section 2) and cure with following surgery has been reported. In advanced cases jaundice and itch, if present, can usually be relieved by a surgical operation in which the obstruction to bile flow is bypassed, allowing the bile to flow into the bowel by another route.

CANCER OF THE PANCREAS

Cancer of the pancreas has been becoming increasingly common in westernised societies over recent years. It is now the third leading cause of cancer death in middle-aged males in the USA. It is more common in males than females, although its cause is unknown. It is becoming increasingly common in smokers and is also more common in heavy drinkers of alcohol. People with diabetes have a somewhat increased risk of developing cancer in the pancreas.

Symptoms and signs

Cancer of the pancreas often involves the bile duct from the liver, which passes through the pancreas. As the cancer grows it commonly blocks the bile duct, obstructing the flow of bile from the liver into the intestine and so causing jaundice. As the obstruction continues, the jaundice becomes a deeper yellow colour. The jaundice is sometimes painless, although there is often pain felt deep in the upper abdomen and passing through to the back. As the jaundice develops, the patient's skin may become very itchy. The liver and gall bladder often become enlarged due to obstruction of the bile duct. Occasionally the cancer can be felt as a lump in the upper abdomen.

Figure 1. Upper abdominal organs showing position of the pancreas (mostly behind the stomach)

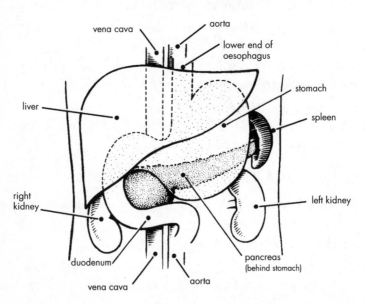

In most patients with cancer of the pancreas, weight loss becomes obvious. It may even be the first feature of this disease. Anorexia (loss of appetite) is usual and diarrhoea may also be present.

Investigations

As the pancreas lies across the back of the upper abdomen behind the stomach and other organs (see Figure 1), it has been one of the more difficult organs to feel or investigate. However, in recent years, improved methods of investigation have been developed which may reveal abnormalities including cancer.

Ultrasound and CT scans have been of some help in detecting earlier cancers, although early detection of the smallest and most potentially curable cancers is still difficult.

Examination of the pancreatic duct using an endoscope passed through the mouth and via the stomach into the duodenum (ERCP examination) has allowed pancreatic secretions to be examined for cancer cells and X-rays to be taken of the duct. These may be helpful in detecting evidence of some pancreatic cancers at an early stage.

As yet, an isotope material suitable and specific for scanning the pancreas has not been available. However, work continues in the search for such a substance. When PET scans become more readily available (see Section 2), it is hoped that they will give considerable help in early detection and diagnosis, and also in showing response to treatments used.

Needle biopsy of any lump in the pancreas is the most useful method of establishing a diagnosis, although this procedure does have risks and is not always reliable.

Treatment

At the time of detection, cancer of the pancreas has usually spread to the liver as well as lymph nodes and cure by surgery is usually not possible. However, occasionally small early cancers can be resected by a major surgical operation with some hope of cure.

To date, treatment by radiotherapy or chemotherapy has been disappointing, although more effective anti-cancer drugs in more effective combinations are constantly being investigated. Present studies include more effective use of intra-arterial chemotherapy as the first measure of an integrated treatment program with radiotherapy and surgery, but a number of difficulties need to be solved before this can be more widely recommended as safe treatment. At this stage, some hope of temporary palliation of symptoms is usually the best that can be achieved.

For those people with jaundice due to pancreatic cancer obstructing the bile duct, relief of the jaundice can usually be achieved by a surgical operation in which the obstruction to the bile duct is bypassed.

CANCER OF THE SMALL INTESTINE

Cancer of the small intestine is rare. The most common of the rare primary malignant tumours of the small intestine are a lymphoma, and a tumour called a carcinoid (cancer-like) tumour. These are rare causes of abdominal pain, bowel bleeding and small bowel obstruction. They are usually treated by a surgical operation in which the tumour is removed with part of the bowel.

Carcinoid tumours may occur anywhere in the alimentary (digestive) tract. That is, they may occur anywhere between the mouth and the anus, but the most common site of a carcinoid tumour is the appendix. Most carcinoids in the appendix (and in fact most small carcinoids) are not malignant. Sometimes when an appendix has been removed, a small carcinoid tumour may be found in it. In most such cases the tumour has been cured by removal of the appendix and further treatment is usually not necessary.

When a carcinoid tumour is found in the small intestine, it is more likely to be larger, more likely to be malignant and may have already spread to the liver. Secondary carcinoids in the liver may release certain biochemical substances that can cause bouts of diarrhoea, flushing of the skin of the face, or wheezing of the lungs. Treatment can be given to control these episodes, but once this tumour has spread into the liver a complete cure is unlikely.

CANCER OF THE LARGE BOWEL

In Western societies the large bowel is the most common site of primary cancer other than skin cancer. In the adult population of the USA (both men and women), bowel cancer is responsible for more deaths than any other cancer. It is occasionally seen in young adults and even in children, but is not commonly seen until after the age of 40 years. Thereafter the incidence rises with age, reaching a peak between 60 and 75 years.

As discussed in Section 1, cancer of the large bowel is most common in societies where the food intake is relatively high in meat and animal fats and relatively low in fibre such as in wholemeal grains, fruit and vegetables.

Polyps in the large bowel also predispose to cancer and, if present, should be removed to avoid the risk of malignant change. People who have had polyps removed should be kept under regular observation in case more develop.

The uncommon hereditary condition, familial polyposis coli, is one in which about half of the members of an affected family are likely to develop multiple polyps. It is a highly pre-malignant condition, and all close blood relatives in an affected family should be kept under regular observation. If polyps are found, the large bowel should be removed to prevent the development of cancer later in life. If this is not done, most people will have developed a bowel cancer by the age of about 40 years.

Other conditions associated with an increased risk of

development of large bowel cancer are the inflammatory bowel disease, granular (Crohn's) colitis, and more especially ulcerative colitis. People with longstanding and extensive ulcerative colitis must be kept under close and regular observation and in some circumstances may be well advised to have the colon removed as a precautionary measure.

Apart from the condition of familial polyposis coli, it has been found that close relatives of a patient with large bowel cancer also have a slightly increased risk of developing a similar cancer. Whether this is mainly due to a truly genetic factor or to similar diet and other habits is uncertain. It is also true that after successful treatment of one large bowel cancer, the patient has a rather greater than average risk of developing a second cancer in the large bowel, although by far the majority of such patients never develop a new cancer. However, regular follow-up observation is desirable for all patients previously treated for bowel cancer, as indeed it is desirable for all patients previously treated for any form of cancer.

Symptoms and signs

The most common symptoms associated with large bowel cancer are a change in bowel habits (constipation or diarrhoea or sometimes alternating constipation and diarrhoea), bleeding from the bowel, and a feeling of incomplete evacuation of the bowel after going to the toilet. In some cases, the sufferer may not notice any symptoms until the cancer has caused bowel obstruction. The first symptoms may thus be symptoms of bowel obstruction, with intermittent griping abdominal pain (colic), constipation and abdominal distension.

Other features of large bowel cancer may be general debility, weight loss, tiredness and lassitude (sometimes due to anaemia) or features of liver enlargement or jaundice due to secondary spread into the liver.

The doctor may be able to feel a lump or localised swelling in the abdomen or, on examination through the anus, a mass in the rectum. There may be evidence of blood in the faeces. In the case of obstructive bowel cancer, evidence of bowel obstruction with abdominal distension or swelling may be found.

Investigations

These are described in Section 2. Investigations that may help in establishing a diagnosis include examination with a sigmoidoscope through the anus. About 50% of large bowel cancers are in the rectum or the lowest part of the colon just above the rectum, and most of these can be seen and biopsied through a sigmoidoscope.

Barium enema screening and X-rays may reveal a cancer, especially if air contrast barium study is used (see Section 2).

If there is no evidence of bowel obstruction and especially if a cancer is suspected in the first part of the large bowel (the caecum), then barium meal studies and X-rays may help in outlining a tumour mass.

Sigmoidoscopic examination, barium enema and barium meal studies may all be done on an outpatient basis. Examination with a modern colonoscope, however, requires heavy sedation or general anaesthesia, but this examination will allow the whole length of the large bowel to be examined visually and for biopsies to be taken from any part of the length of the colon. A day in hospital is usually required for this examination.

Blood studies are carried out for evidence of anaemia and for evidence of changes in biochemistry of the blood or impaired liver function. One particular blood test useful for diagnosis, management and to study progress of a patient with large bowel cancer is the CEA (carcino-embrionic antigen) test. This is an immune reaction test that is usually strongly positive in people with large bowel cancer and becomes negative after successful treatment. If it becomes positive again after treatment, it may suggest recurrence of the cancer.

Liver isotope scans or CT scans may also be taken to look for any evidence of secondary liver cancer.

Treatment

The only way to cure a large bowel cancer is by a surgical operation in which that part of the bowel containing the cancer is excised together with draining lymph nodes into which the cancer may have spread. In most cases the bowel is joined together again and the patient can return to normal life.

When the cancer is in the lower rectum it may be necessary to remove the anus as well as the rectum; an opening for the lower bowel is made in the abdominal wall to allow evacuation of faeces. This opening is called a colostomy. The patient learns to wear a bag over the colostomy, and the bowel empties at regular intervals into the bag. The patient learns to empty the bag at convenient times and gradually learns to live an active and virtually normal life.

Membership of a **colostomy club**, which has branches in many large cities, is available for all people who have a colostomy. This club offers support and advice on learning to live with a colostomy and the other social adjustments that may worry these patients.

In the hands of a good surgeon, an early operation will cure about half the patients with large bowel cancer. With or without a colostomy, most of these then return to normal life.

If a cancer first appears with a bowel obstruction, it may be necessary to perform a temporary colostomy operation to relieve the obstruction. Usually the cancer is removed at a further surgical operation three or four weeks later, and the colostomy is closed, resulting in a return to a normal passage of bowel actions.

Follow-up care

As for all patients who have had treatment for cancer, regular follow-up consultations and care are required for patients who have had a bowel cancer removed. There is always a risk of secondary cancer showing up in the liver or elsewhere and there may be a risk of another cancer developing which can be effectively treated if detected while still small. In the case of bowel cancer, any secondary cancer usually shows up within two years; it is uncommon for it to appear after five years. If the patient has been followed up for five years without evidence of recurrence, he or she is usually considered to be cured.

If the cancer has spread to the liver, cure is not possible except in occasional cases where there is only one lump in the liver and this lump can be resected in a surgical operation, or more occasionally when there are two or three lumps in the liver but only in a part of the liver that can be safely resected.

Treatment with radiotherapy or chemotherapy has been disappointing for large bowel cancer, although secondary spread to the liver can sometimes be temporarily controlled by the use of anti-cancer drugs. Control is best achieved if the drugs are infused directly into the artery that supplies blood to the liver. The recent development of an implantable pump to continuously infuse cytotoxic drugs into the artery supplying blood to the liver has shown encouraging results as far as improving the patient's quality of life and life expectancy are concerned, but as yet will still not achieve total cure.

Different combinations of anti-cancer drugs given in different treatment schedules with or without infusion pumps are under study in many world cancer centres. Although it is clear that best results are achieved when the drugs are given into the artery that supplies blood to the liver, as yet there are a number of problems to be solved before this form of treatment can be recommended for general use.

CANCER OF THE ANUS

Cancer of the anus is not common, but may present as a lump, an ulcer, bleeding or pain in the anal region. Sometimes it may develop in a pre-existing benign lesion such as a papilloma (a fern-like growth from the bowel lining), a patch of leukoplakia (white patch) or in a longstanding anal fissure (a crack in the wall of the opening of the anus).

Most cancers of the anus are similar in type to SCC of skin, but behave more aggressively in that they tend to spread to lymph nodes in the groin or in the pelvis at an earlier stage and often require radical treatment to achieve the best chances of cure.

Treatment

A biopsy is taken to confirm the presence of cancer and the type of cancer. Treatment may then be by local surgery or radio-therapy for small early cancers, or radical surgery including excision of the rectum and anus for more advanced cancers. Radical removal of draining lymph nodes from the groin will be required if these nodes appear to be involved.

Attempts at improving results and at reducing the need for radical surgery by first reducing the cancers with pre-operative chemotherapy are being carried out in some centres. Results of such combined and integrated treatment programs have been encouraging, so that in some specialised cancer centres integrated treatment has become standard practice for advanced cancers.

Cancers of the head and neck

Cancers of the lips, mouth, tongue, nasal cavity, the paranasal air sinuses, throat, larynx and pharynx (the passage at the back of the nose and mouth) constitute about 5% of all cancers recorded in the USA. European, Canadian and Australasian figures are similar. Most of these cancers are similar in type to SCCs of the skin but tend to behave in a more malignant or a more aggressive fashion. As a rule, the further away the cancers are from the lips the more aggressively they behave. Cancers of the lips are more aggressive than skin cancers. That is, they tend to grow more rapidly and have a greater tendency to spread to draining lymph nodes at an earlier stage. Cancers of the floor of the mouth, the anterior two-thirds of the tongue and palate are more aggressive than cancers of the lips. Cancers of the back of the tongue, in the region of the tonsils and pharynx and upper air passages are the most aggressive of all. Cancers of the vocal cords of the larynx are an exception to this rule. Most remain localised to the vocal cords, with no evidence of spread when they first cause symptoms: most are readily curable at that stage.

These cancers are all more common in smokers than in non-smokers. It has been estimated that cancers in the mouth and throat are about six times more common in smokers, and this is increased to about fifteen times if the smokers are also heavy drinkers of alcohol. Other pre-malignant conditions that predispose to cancer in the mouth include leukoplakia, papillomata, and chronic irritation from such causes as ill-fitting dentures or jagged teeth (see Section 1). Cancer of the buccal mucosa (cheek lining) is common in India and South-East Asia, where betel nut chewing is a common practice. It is especially common in people who mix betel nut with tobacco leaf or lime and hold the mixture in the cheek pouch.

CANCERS OF THE LIPS

Cancers of the lips are more obvious than cancers further back in the mouth or throat and for this reason they are usually diagnosed at an earlier and more curable stage. They may develop as a thickening in an area of hyperkeratosis (sun damage) of the lip – usually the lower lip. They tend to ulcerate and possibly bleed or may form a lump. They may spread to lymph nodes under the jaw and in the sides of the neck and form small lumps in these places.

A biopsy is taken to confirm the diagnosis and thereafter treatment is usually by surgical excision with good results both cosmetically (in appearance) and in eventual cure rates. Radiotherapy may also be used with good results.

For larger cancers of the lips, either radical surgery removing a large part of the lip (with some form of plastic or reconstructive surgery to fashion a new lip) or radiotherapy may be used, and the chances of cure are still quite good.

If hard, enlarged lymph nodes are present either when the patient is first seen or at a later follow-up visit to the doctor, then these are best treated by surgical excision – a block dissection (an operation to remove all lymph nodes in one block of tissue).

Occasionally, a patient first consults a doctor when the cancer is very large and possibly the whole of the lip is involved with cancer. In these patients, considerable success can be achieved with chemotherapy, preferably given at first by infusion into the arteries that supply blood to the region (to reduce the size of the tumour), followed by treatment with radiotherapy or surgery or both. Such treatment should be done only in specialist clinics with special experience, equipment and skills, and is not necessary for small cancers that can be readily cured by operation or by radiotherapy (see Section 2).

CANCERS OF THE FLOOR OF THE MOUTH (UNDER THE TONGUE), ANTERIOR TWO-THIRDS OF THE TONGUE AND BUCCAL MUCOSA (INSIDE THE CHEEK)

These cancers are more aggressive than lip cancers (i.e. they grow more rapidly and spread more rapidly), and enlargement of lymph nodes containing secondary spread of cancer is rather common.

These cancers are usually first noticed as an ulcer or a lump, sometimes by a dentist, before the patient has become aware of any problem. Other common features are bleeding or localised soreness. They tend to be on the surface at first, but soon invade locally, with firm thickness and induration surrounding the lump or ulcer. They usually become quite tender. Diagnosis is confirmed by taking a small piece of tissue as a biopsy for examination under the microscope.

Most cancers are treated by surgical excision or radiotherapy. Lymph nodes are best treated by surgical excision of all lymph nodes in the region (block dissection).

For larger cancers in the floor of the mouth, anterior two-thirds of tongue, and possibly in the cheek, treatment by chemotherapy (*Induction or neoadjuvant chemotherapy* – see Section 2) preferably given by regional intra-arterial infusion followed by radiotherapy or surgery or both gives best results in some specialist clinics. By these combined treatment methods, cures can now be achieved in patients with advanced cancers that until recently were considered incurable or possibly curable only by most radical surgery. Such treatments require special skills, equipment and experience and should only be carried out in specialist cancer centres (see Section 2).

CANCER IN THE POSTERIOR THIRD OF THE TONGUE, TONSILLAR REGION AND PHARYNX

People with these cancers may present with an ulcer, a lump in the throat or tongue or sometimes with a constant sore throat that has not responded to medical treatment including antibiotics. Sometimes patients will first notice a lump in the side of the neck which is an enlarged, hard lymph node containing secondary cancer. Diagnosis may appear to be obvious but must be confirmed by biopsy.

Except for small cancers in this region, most are not curable by surgery. Radiotherapy is likely to cure only small cancers, although it may offer good temporary palliation to people with large cancers.

Most people with these cancers do not attend a doctor or clinic until the cancer is advanced and the chances of cure by surgery or radiotherapy are not good. Most will be heavy smokers and many will also be heavy drinkers of alcohol and will not notice symptoms until the tumours are advanced. In any case, these cancers are aggressive and tend to grow and invade locally and spread into lymph nodes in one or both sides of the neck at a relatively early stage.

Radical surgery will cure some of these patients and radiotherapy may cure others and offer palliation to the majority. However, the experience of this author and an increasing number of international experts in combined integrated treatment methods, is that best results are achieved by induction chemotherapy via intra-arterial infusion followed by radiotherapy or surgery or both.

CANCERS OF THE POST-NASAL SPACE (BACK OF THE NOSE)

These cancers are most common in adult Chinese people, especially those from the Kwangtung province of China. Sons and daughters of people from Kwangtung also have an increased incidence of this cancer even though they may never have lived in China.

Blood tests show that this cancer is most common in people who have been infected with the Epstein-Barr virus: their blood usually has a high level of Epstein-Barr virus antibodies. If the Epstein-Barr test is high before treatment and returns to normal after treatment, it indicates that treatment has been successful and the patient has probably been cured.

Symptoms and signs

People with post-nasal space cancer may present with symptoms of a blocked nose, nasal or post-nasal discharge of mucus, pus or bloodstained material or, alternatively, they sometimes first notice a lump in the side of the neck. The lump is due to secondary cancer in a lymph node. Sometimes lymph nodes on both sides of the neck are involved.

The cancer may sometimes be seen with a mirror in the back of the throat, but diagnosis is made by taking a biopsy from the back of the nose or sometimes by removing for pathological examination an enlarged lymph node from the neck.

Occasionally the cancer invades bones at the base of the skull or the cranial nerves that pass from the brain through the base of the skull and into the neck. Special X-rays (tomograms) or CT scans may be taken to look for evidence of bone involvement.

Treatment

Cancer in the back of the nose is not accessible to surgery. It is usually treated by radiotherapy with better than a 50% chance of cure provided the cancer has not spread into lymph nodes in the neck or invaded bone behind the nose at the base of the skull. If lymph nodes in the neck are involved, the chance of cure by radiotherapy alone is reduced (possibly only 30–40%) and considerably less if nodes on both sides of the neck are involved. The possibility of improving results by first giving a course of chemotherapy by intravenous injection before radiotherapy is currently under investigation. Such combined integrated chemotherapy and radiotherapy is giving better results in the treatment of advanced cancers, especially if lymph nodes are involved.

If bone at the base of the skull is invaded by cancer, the chance of cure by any means is poor.

CANCER OF THE LARYNX

This cancer is most common in smokers, and especially in smokers who are also heavy drinkers. It is more common in men than women. The most common site for cancer in the larynx is on a vocal cord. Cancers of the vocal cord usually cause a hoarseness or change in the voice when they are quite small and are therefore usually diagnosed early. They can be seen and biopsied through a laryngoscope and if treated early either by radiotherapy or by surgery (in which the cord is removed), the results of treatment are good. About 90% are cured.

If neglected until the cancer has grown from the vocal cord into surrounding tissues, the chances of cure by simple surgery or radiotherapy are much reduced.

For more advanced laryngeal cancers that have spread to the walls of the larynx or spread into lymph nodes in the neck, or cancers that have recurred after previous radiotherapy, the best chance of cure is by radical surgery in which the larynx is removed, possibly together with all draining lymph nodes (an operation called a radical laryngectomy). Cancers in the larynx that develop above or below the vocal cords are usually more advanced when they are first diagnosed than cancers on a vocal cord. They also tend to be more aggressive and for this reason are often treated by combined radiotherapy and laryngectomy.

After removal of the larynx, the chance of cure is reasonably good, but the patient (usually a male) is left with an opening of his windpipe in the lower neck (tracheostomy). Without a larynx he cannot speak normally, but most patients learn a form of oesophageal speech. By this method they can be taught to swallow air and use air regurgitated from the stomach to make sounds and words. Alternatively, a mechanical vibrator powered by a small battery can be applied to the throat muscles to make speech which sounds rather like the artificial voice of a robot or computer.

The **Lost Cords club** is a group for people who have lost their larynx and support each other in learning to speak and in other social, health and mechanical problems. As for the mastectomy club (for women who have had a breast removed) and the colostomy club (for patients with a colostomy), there are branches in many big cities. The club supports people who have had a laryngectomy by helping them to adjust to changed circumstances. It also helps patients in learning to speak so that they can live a relatively normal life again.

SALIVARY GLAND CANCERS

The salivary glands are located about the mouth and secrete saliva into the mouth, especially to prepare food for digestion. There are three major and many minor salivary glands on each side of the face.

The largest salivary gland is the parotid gland, situated partly in front of and below the ear and behind the jaw. This is the salivary gland in which both benign and malignant tumours develop most commonly. The second largest major salivary gland is the submandibular gland under the jaw and the third major salivary gland is the sublingual gland in the floor of the mouth under the tongue. The many small minor salivary glands are in the mucous membrane (lining) of the tongue, lips, palate, cheek and pharynx.

Cancers of the salivary glands are usually first noticed as a lump, most commonly just in front of or below the ear. As the cancer enlarges, it may invade and destroy an important nerve, the facial nerve, which passes through the parotid gland. Damage to the facial nerve causes weakness of the muscles of that side of the face, resulting in an inability to close the eye or move the corner of the mouth properly. There may be obvious loss of facial expression due to paralysis of the muscles on that side of the face. These cancers most often develop in middle-aged or older adults. They enlarge locally and tend to spread to local lymph nodes in front of the ear and in the upper part of the neck. Occasionally cancers develop from a pre-existing benign tumour in the parotid gland that may have been present for years, known as a mixed parotid tumour or pleomorphic adenoma.

Treatment of cancers of the parotid gland is usually by removal at a surgical operation. With small cancers it may be possible to save the facial nerve, but with larger cancers it is likely that the facial nerve will be involved and will need to be removed. If lymph nodes are found to be enlarged, they are usually removed in the same block of tissue with the parotid gland. Post-operative radiotherapy is often given in view of the risk of local recurrence of these cancers.

Cancers in the submandibular and sublingual salivary glands are not common, but when present they tend to spread early to lymph nodes and are best treated by surgical excision of the whole of the gland, together with any involved lymph nodes. Salivary gland tumours occasionally occur in the minor salivary glands, either in the tongue, in the cheeks, lips or elsewhere. Wide surgical excision is required for treatment, as the chances of local recurrence are high unless a lot of tissue around the lump is removed. If there is any doubt that the cancer has been totally removed, then radiotherapy may also be given after the operation.

The use of chemotherapy in the treatment of salivary gland tumours is not yet established. It has been used with limited success in the treatment of cancers that have recurred after surgery. The use of chemotherapy before surgical excision of salivary gland tumours is under investigation, but as yet it is uncertain as to whether results will be significantly improved by this technique.

CANCER OF THE THYROID GLAND

The thyroid gland lies across the lower part of the neck, with one lobe on either side of the trachea (or windpipe) and on the lower part of the larynx (voice box). The thyroid gland uses iodine to make a hormone called thyroxine which is essential for normal body function.

Enlargement of the thyroid gland is called a goitre, and multiple cysts and other lumps may develop in some goitres. This process is usually due to a shortage of iodine in the food. A lumpy goitre is known as a multinodular goitre.

Occasionally one of the lumps in a multinodular goitre will become malignant and form a cancer, but more often a cancer develops as a single lump in an otherwise apparently normal thyroid gland.

Thus cancer of the thyroid is usually first noticed as a single lump in the thyroid gland, most often just to one or other side of the midline in the lower part of the neck. It may occasionally develop in a goitre as one lump that enlarges and becomes more obvious and more hard.

Investigations

An isotope scan is a useful investigation for thyroid cancer. A scan of the thyroid is taken after injection of a very small dose of radioactive iodine into a vein (see Section 2) and will usually show a 'cold nodule', that is, part of the thyroid gland that is replaced by cancer does not concentrate the iodine and appears clear on the scan. However, cysts and some other lumps also show up as 'cold nodules'; to make a diagnosis, the lump should be biopsied. This may sometimes be done by needle aspiration of fluid or cells from the lump. Alternatively the diagnosis is more certain if the lump is surgically excised and examined under a microscope. Frozen section examination (see Section 2) may then allow the surgeon to proceed with further surgery if the lump proves to be a cancer.

There are three main types of thyroid cancer.

The most common of the thyroid cancers (more than 60%) is the least malignant. This is called a **papillary** cancer, and occurs three times more commonly in women than men. This cancer often occurs in young people, occasionally teenagers or even children.

Papillary cancer may be present in different parts of the thyroid gland at the same time and may spread to nearby draining lymph nodes, but usually does not spread further until very late in the disease. For this reason, removal of the whole of the thyroid gland together with any enlarged lymph nodes will usually cure the patient. After total removal of the thyroid gland the patient thereafter must take thyroid or thyroxine tablets by mouth, as thyroxine is essential for normal body function.

The second most common type of thyroid cancer more commonly affects adults of middle age and is called **follicular** cancer.

It, too, usually presents as a lump in the thyroid gland and is usually not diagnosed with certainty until the lump has been removed surgically and examined under the microscope.

These cancers tend to be present in one lobe of the thyroid gland only and have a greater tendency to spread by the bloodstream to bone, lungs or liver rather than by lymphatics to lymph nodes. These cancers often more closely resemble normal thyroid tissue than do the other thyroid cancers and although they usually appear as 'cold nodules' (areas of no function) in radio-iodine scans, they may sometimes scan as normal thyroid tissue or even rarely as hyperactive 'hot nodules' (areas with increased thyroid function).

Because of their tendency to involve one lobe of the thyroid gland only, they are usually treated by removal of the involved half of the thyroid gland, leaving the other half to carry out normal thyroid function and production of thyroxine.

Secondary cancers may be treated by surgical excision (if in lymph nodes) by radiotherapy or by radio-active iodine treatment. Chemotherapy is also sometimes used in the treatment of secondary cancers.

The third broad type of thyroid cancer is **anaplastic cancer**. As this is the most dangerous form of thyroid cancer, it is fortunate that it is also the least common. It tends to affect older people and may grow rapidly, presenting as an enlarging lump or enlarging swelling of the whole of the thyroid gland. It may press on the trachea (windpipe) and make breathing difficult. This cancer is virtually not curable by surgery and is best palliated by radiotherapy or sometimes by chemotherapy.

The thyroid gland is occasionally the site of other primary malignant tumours such as medullary cancer, lymphoma, sarcoma or even secondary cancers from primary cancer elsewhere, but these are uncommon forms of thyroid malignancy.

Cancers of the female sexual organs

CANCER OF THE UTERUS

There are two distinct types of cancer of the uterus – squamous cell carcinoma (SCC) of the cervix or opening of the uterus and endometrial or glandular cancer (adenocarcinoma) of the lining of the cavity of the uterus (the body of the uterus). SCC of the cervix is more common.

CANCER OF THE CERVIX

This cancer is rare in women who have not had children but is more common in women who have had several children, particularly if sexual activity started early in life. Prostitutes and women who have had many male partners also have an increased risk of developing this cancer. Erosions and inflammation of the cervix are predisposing factors. Infection with a sexually transmitted virus, the papilloma virus, can also predispose to later development of cervical cancer.

The earliest changes associated with this cancer are most frequently present in women between the ages of 30 and 40 years. Usually at this age there are no symptoms, but there may be a little blood staining from the vagina between periods, especially after intercourse.

Cancers of the cervix tend to develop slowly but can usually be detected by routine cervical screening examination (the Papanicolaou or cervical smear test described in Section 2) in which abnormal (dysplastic) or frankly malignant cells may be found. An annual routine cervical smear test of women at risk will usually detect these cancers early and at a very curable stage.

Sometimes the cancers cannot be seen on visual examination of the cervix but at other times may be seen as a reddish, eroded, ulcerated or possibly bleeding lesion. A biopsy is taken for pathological examination to confirm the diagnosis.

**Figure 2. Female pelvis showing position of female genital organs
The ovaries are on either side of the uterus**

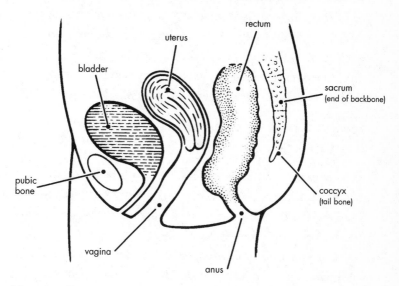

Very small early cancers may be treated by surgical removal of the cervix only, especially in women who wish to have more babies. Larger invasive cancers are best treated by removal of the uterus (total hysterectomy).

If cancer of the cervix has not been diagnosed until it is more advanced, there is a risk that it may have spread to lymph nodes, especially the lymph nodes in the pelvis. This situation is more likely to be found in women of more than 40 years of age who have not had regular cervical smear test examinations. These women often complain of some bleeding and discharge between periods. If an advanced, ulcerating or fungating cancer is present, it should be obvious on examination of the cervix. Surrounding tissues such as the ureters (the tubes that pass urine from the kidneys to the bladder) or the rectum may become involved as well as the local draining lymph nodes in the pelvis. Such advanced cancers are usually treated by radiotherapy, possibly followed by surgery. Chemotherapy has also been used, but to date success has been limited. The most promising use of chemo-therapy to cure this cancer is as the first step in an integrated treatment program – particularly if given by infusion into the arteries supplying blood to the uterus and pelvis ('induction' treatment) – followed by radiotherapy, then by surgery. Such combined integrated treatment is not necessary for early cancers, but does give better prospects for cure of advanced cancers.

CANCER OF THE BODY OF THE UTERUS (ENDOMETRIAL CANCER)

These cancers tend to occur in older women, usually after the menopause. It is believed that change in female sex hormones and especially an imbalance of hormones may contribute to development of these cancers.

The most common feature is bleeding and blood-stained discharge after the menopause. The uterus is usually found to be enlarged. To make a diagnosis the doctor performs a curettage and sends the specimens removed for microscopic examination.

Treatment of cancer of the body of the uterus is usually by total removal of the uterus (total hysterectomy) with removal of ovaries as well as lymph nodes in the pelvis. For advanced cancers, radiotherapy is often given first followed by hysterectomy.

Like most cancers, treatment at an early stage will allow good results, but for more advanced cancers results of treatment are often disappointing.

If endometrial cancer has spread to other tissues or organs it will often respond to hormone treatment (large-dose proges-terone therapy), but a long-term cure is unlikely. Studies are being made of combined integrated treatment using intra-arterial chemotherapy first as 'induction' treatment followed by radio-therapy and/or surgery (see Section 2) but whether or not such treatment will achieve significantly better results is as yet uncertain.

CHORIOCARCINOMA

Although a choriocarcinoma starts and grows in the uterus, it is not strictly a cancer of the uterus. A choriocarcinoma is best considered as a cancer of an abnormal pregnancy.

After conception, very occasionally an abnormal growth of tissue develops instead of a normal foetus and placenta. If the foetus does not develop and the placenta grows as a group of cyst-like structures something like a bunch of grapes, this is called a hydatidiform mole.

Sometimes the cells of a hydatidiform mole develop into an invasive cancer that is called a choriocarcinoma. Occasionally choriocarcinoma will develop in association with a foetus, usually abnormal, which is aborted spontaneously, or even with an otherwise normal pregnancy. However, most in fact are in association with a hydatidiform mole, usually in women over 40 years of age.

In the past, choriocarcinoma spread widely and rapidly through the mother's body and was a fatal form of cancer. Nowadays the condition is treated by emptying the uterus of its contents (a curette) and giving cytotoxic chemotherapy. This is one of the success stories of modern chemotherapy, as chorio-carcinoma, almost 100% fatal about 30 years ago, is now curable in 80% or more cases.

CANCER OF THE OVARY

The ovaries are the source of a greater variety of tumours, both benign and malignant, than any other body organ. This is prob-ably because of the nature of the ovaries as organs with a func-tion of undergoing monthly cyclic changes to produce eggs or ova for potential development into new tissues of a foetus. They may also produce tumours that excrete hormones which may affect body development and function.

Cancers of the ovary may be solid, cystic or contain a mixture of solid and cystic elements. They tend to cause no symptoms early in their development and so are often quite advanced when first diagnosed.

Symptoms and signs

Cancers of the ovary usually cause a swelling in the pelvis and lower abdomen. The swelling may have been noticed by the patient or may be found on examination by a doctor. They may sometimes cause local discomfort or pain. If they produce hormones, the first evidence may be due to hormonal changes such as premature cessation of menstruation and loss of feminine features with a development of male characteristics such as growth of hair on the face or deepening of the voice. Sometimes generalised abdominal swelling may also be noticed, due either to a huge tumour or to fluid in the abdominal cavity (ascites).

Any rapidly enlarging swelling on an ovary, especially if it is solid or contains a mixture of cystic and solid elements, must be regarded with suspicion as likely to be malignant (cancer).

Investigations

A doctor will carry out examination of the pelvis and pelvic structures by examining the lower abdomen, the vagina and rectum, but if this examination is not adequate the patient may be admitted to hospital for examination under a general anaesthetic.

Abdominal X-rays or CT scans may help, but ultrasound examination is the least harmful examination, especially in young women, and usually the most helpful.

Laparoscopy or culdoscopy (see Section 2) may allow the surgeon or gynaecologist to see the contents of the pelvis, especially the ovaries.

Usually the diagnosis of cancer cannot be established with

certainty until an operation (laparotomy) has been carried out and a biopsy specimen of any suspicious lesion has been examined under the microscope.

Treatment

The best treatment of ovarian cancer is by surgical removal of the ovaries. As the other ovary and sometimes other pelvic organs may also contain cancer, it is usual to remove both ovaries as well as the uterus and tubes and any other involved tissue. Operation is followed by radiotherapy to the pelvis. If the cancer cannot be removed, the patient is usually treated by radiotherapy.

Chemotherapy is often effective in controlling widespread secondary cancers for a worthwhile period (possibly some years) but long-term cure is unlikely. Combinations of local chemotherapy (by intra-arterial infusion and/or into the peritoneal cavity) with radiotherapy and/or surgery are presently under study in specialist clinics, but it is not yet certain whether these techniques of integrated treatment will achieve significantly better results with safety.

Prevention

As cancers sometimes develop from benign tumours of the ovary and the ovaries have little function in post-menopausal women, it is usually advisable to remove both ovaries of women over 40 years when treating a benign ovarian tumour. Gynaecologists also often advise removal of ovaries as a preventive measure when they perform hysterectomy (removal of the uterus) in women over the age of 40 years.

The ovaries are commonly a site for development of secondary cancer from a primary cancer elsewhere. Cancer of the breast, stomach, bowel and melanoma frequently spread to ovaries. These are removed if there is no apparent cancer anywhere else, otherwise treatment given will depend upon the best treatment for the type of cancer concerned and where it came from.

CANCER OF THE VULVA

Like cancer of the anus, cancer of the vulva is a rather aggressive form of skin cancer, usually of the SCC type. Most occur in women of post-menopausal age. This cancer is often preceded by a long history of irritation or discomfort of the vulva, possibly with a local blood-stained discharge. There may be a pre-malignant condition of leukoplakia or a chronic rash. Previous infection with the sexually transmitted papilloma virus may be responsible for some cases.

In the more advanced disease there may be an ulcer, a lump or a cauliflower-like growth. Spread to lymph nodes in one or both groins is likely to be present in about half of the patients.

Diagnosis is established by biopsy and treatment is usually by wide and radical surgical excision, most often with satisfactory results, most patients being cured. Pre-malignant conditions are also best treated by surgical excision to prevent cancer developing.

For very advanced cases, radiotherapy offers palliative relief. Integrated treatment using intra-arterial induction chemotherapy followed by radiotherapy and/or surgery is presently under study in some specialised centres. As yet it is not known whether better long-term results will be achieved with safety.

Cancer of the male sexual organs

CANCER OF THE TESTIS

Testicular tumours are not common, but when they do occur they are almost always malignant. Most occur in young adult males between the ages of 20 and 40 years.

Figure 3. Male pelvis showing position of the prostate gland

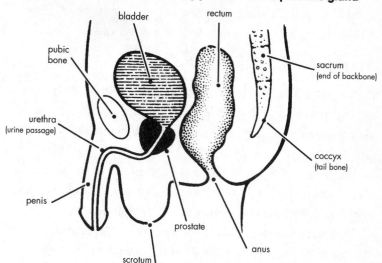

There are no known causes of testicular cancer, although they are distinctly more likely to occur in testes that have not descended from the abdomen, where they develop, into the scrotum where they should be present at birth. If both testes are not present in the scrotum of infant boys, surgical operation may be required to place the testes in their normal position. This may reduce the risk of development of cancer later in life, after puberty.

Symptoms and signs

Cancer of the testis is usually found as a painless and non-tender swelling of a testis, although occasionally the swelling is tender and possibly painful. Occasionally no swelling is noticed in the testis until there is evidence of secondary spread of a cancer. These may be noticed as a mass of enlarged and sometimes tender lymph nodes in the abdomen, enlarged lymph nodes in the neck (usually the left side) or as secondary cancers in lungs seen in a chest X-ray. Occasionally the first evidence of a testicular cancer may be swelling of a man's breasts due to changes in his hormones. In other patients the first evidence may be of general debility, anorexia (loss of appetite) and weight loss.

Investigations

If a swelling of a testis is likely to be cancer, investigations are carried out to look for evidence of secondary spread. Radio-isotope scans (using gallium), excretory urograms (IVP X-rays) or CT scans have all been described in Section 2. These may be helpful in detecting any enlarged lymph nodes in the abdomen. Chest X-rays may help detect secondary cancers in lungs or in lymph nodes in the chest (mediastinal lymph nodes).

To confirm diagnosis of cancer, an operation is recommended to allow the testis to be examined and biopsied. Usually a frozen section technique is used while the patient is still under the anaesthetic so that the operation of orchidectomy (removal of the testis) can be carried out immediately if cancer is confirmed.

Treatment

Cancer of a testis is treated by surgical removal of the testis and radiotherapy to draining lymph nodes in the abdomen or any other lymph nodes likely to be involved. It is possible to lead a normal sex life and to father children with only one testis.

If the cancer is widespread into the lungs or elsewhere, encouraging results are being achieved with chemotherapy in increasing numbers of patients because most testicular cancers are sensitive to chemotherapy.

CANCER OF THE PROSTATE GLAND

Cancer of the prostate is uncommon before the age of 50 years, but is the most common cancer in men over 65 years and becoming increasingly common.

Its cause is unknown, but its association with old age is

illustrated by the fact that 75% of men over the age of 90 years have microscopic evidence of at least early prostatic cancer. This cancer is less common in some countries such as Asian and Oriental countries than it is in Western countries. It is likely that differences in diet may play a part, as prostate cancer is less common in communities that have a predominantly vegetarian diet rather than a diet high in animal products.

Recent studies have indicated that diets with a high content of legumes such as soy beans may be protective, and it could be that the high content of naturally occurring hormones (the phytoestrogens) is at least partly responsible.

Symptoms and signs

The most common symptom of prostatic cancer is difficulty passing urine. Non-malignant enlargement of the prostate (prostate hypertrophy) is most often the cause of urinary difficulty, but prostatic cancer is also a common cause of this trouble, especially in older men.

Sometimes the first evidence of cancer of the prostate is due to secondary cancers either in bone (causing bone pain or fractures) or in the liver (causing liver enlargement). Secondary cancers in the lower vertebral column (back bone) or pelvis may cause pressure on a sciatic nerve that passes into the leg, causing severe pain in the back and leg called sciatica. Sciatica is more often caused by other diseases, but sometimes it is the first evidence of a cancer of the prostate.

Investigations

The prostate gland can be felt by the examining finger when a doctor does a PR (per rectal) examination. That is, a gloved finger is passed through the anus into the rectum and the prostate gland can be felt in front of the finger (see Figure 3). Cancer in the prostate feels like a hard lump in the prostate or sometimes the whole of the prostate gland may feel hard and rigid. A biopsy may be taken with a needle passed through the skin in front of the anus and guided by a finger in the rectum.

Ultrasound is now used with special equipment which is passed through the anus into the rectum. Ultrasound will show any lumps in the prostate and any general prostate enlargement. Biopsies are best taken with a special punch or needle during this examination to discover whether any of the lumps are cancer.

X-rays will be taken for evidence of secondary spread into bones. These usually show up as sclerotic (dense white) areas in the bone. Chest X-rays may show evidence of secondary cancers in the lungs, in lymph nodes in the chest, or even in the ribs. Isotope bone scans are also valuable in showing evidence of secondary bone cancer.

Blood studies may show evidence of anaemia due to secondary bone cancer destroying the blood-forming cells in bone marrow. Cancer of the prostate may also cause an elevation of an enzyme in blood called acid phosphatase, and if bone is destroyed by secondary tumours, an enzyme released from the bone called alkaline phosphatase may also be elevated. The prescence or absence of these enzymes in blood tests will give an indication of the presence or absence of cancer or of secondaries in bone.

Obstruction by the cancer to the flow of urine may cause infection in the bladder and possibly in the kidneys. The urine and blood are examined for evidence of infection in urine and for evidence of damage to the kidneys.

In recent years a new blood test, the **PSA screening test**, has been developed that indicates whether there is likely to be an abnormality in the prostate. This is a special immunological test that is now commonly used in men over the age of 60 years to help find those with early prostate cancer which can be effectively treated by operation. A raised PSA test does not necessarily indicate that cancer is present but it does indicate the need for further investigations, possibly including ultrasound study and biopsies.

Treatment and treatment controversies

Nowhere in the field of cancer treatment is there more confusion than is the case with prostate cancer. The PSA screening test has led to investigation and diagnosis of prostate cancer in increasing numbers of middle-aged and elderly males. Yet even if a biopsy diagnosis of cancer is confirmed it is estimated that only about one in four of those cancers will grow in a malignant fashion and spread to tissues beyond the prostate in such a way that it is likely to cause the patient's death. There is as yet no way of identifying those cancers that are likely to spread. Most prostate cancers are slow growing and even after many years may show no evidence of spread, but some will spread to such places as lungs, liver and especially to bones where they are likely to form painful secondaries and lead to the death of the patient. Appropriate early treatment will cure most patients but all treatments have serious side-effects and it is not possible at this stage to determine which patients will benefit from treatment and who might be as well left without treatment.

The most unavoidable and distressing of side-effects is impotence. This occurs in more than half of the patients whether treated by total prostatectomy (surgical removal of the whole prostate gland) or by radiotherapy. Treatments available at present are often effective for impotence resulting from prostatectomy, but when hormone treatment is used to treat secondaries, either by giving female hormones (oestrogens) or by orchidectomy (castration) or both, permanent impotence is virtually inevitable.

Although controversial, the following are standard treatments that should be considered and discussed between a patient and his medical advisors.

For small cancers apparently confined to the prostate, total surgical removal of the prostate gland, possibly with removal of adjacent lymph nodes, should result in cure. This may be the best treatment for men who are reasonably young and fit.

Alternatively, obstruction to the flow of urine may be relieved by a TUR (trans-urethral resection) in which an instrument (resectoscope) is passed into the urethra through the penis and some of the enlarged prostate is cut away to relieve obstruction. Specimens of the tissue are sent for microscopic examination.

Cancer of the prostate will often respond to radiotherapy, which is often used to treat both primary prostatic cancer and a limited number of painful secondary deposits in bone.

Hormone treatment is also used, especially for more wide-spread cancer. Cancer of the prostate is sensitive to the female hormone called oestrogen. Patients with incurable prostatic cancer are often given effective palliative relief by treatment with oestrogen. An alternative treatment likely to give similar response is to remove the source of male hormones, i.e. to remove the testes. Bilateral orchidectomy (removal of both testes) may be combined with oestrogen therapy for best pallia-tion (relief of symptoms). Patients must be informed of the likely side-effects of oestrogen. Some patients may feel nauseated, many will develop some enlargement and tenderness of the breasts and there is also a slightly increased risk of deep vein thrombosis (blood clots in the legs). Desire for sexual activity will be reduced and there may be complete impotence. However, as oestrogen is effective in giving relief in about 80% of cases, the risk of side-effects is usually well justified.

There have been few studies of the use of cytotoxic chemo-therapy in treatment of prostate cancer. In general, early cancers can be well treated by operation and secondary cancer usually responds well to hormone treatment. These cancers are slow growing so that palliative chemotherapy, with all its side-effects (more toxic than hormone therapy), is not advised, especially in these older age group patients.

Prostatic cancer will respond to treatment with some cytotoxic agents, but these are normally only used in patients whose cancer no longer responds to hormones. Hormones are more reliable, more effective and less toxic than cytotoxic agents in treating this cancer. There is, however, some recent evidence that prostate cancer will respond to concentrated intra-arterial chemotherapy. Studies are now being done in Germany to determine whether better results can be expected from using regional cytotoxic chemotherapy before surgery in treating patients with locally advanced prostate cancers or whether regional chemotherapy used before radiotherapy might make the operation unnecessary in some patients. It is not yet possible to state whether these new approaches will be effective.

Cancers of the bladder and kidneys

BLADDER CANCER

Cancer of the bladder is found to be increased in industrial workers who are exposed to aniline dyes and certain other chemical compounds. It has long been known to be more common in some countries, such as along the Nile valley in Egypt, where parasitic diseases affecting the bladder are more common. It is also increased in smokers. Cancer may also develop in a benign cauliflower-like tumour of the bladder known as a papilloma. Some patients have several small papillomas in the bladder wall and any one of these can change to a bladder cancer if not treated.

The most common symptom of bladder cancer is blood in the urine (haematuria). The blood may be intermittent at first but becomes more constant as the tumour grows and invades the bladder wall. At a later stage there may be discomfort in passing urine (dysuria) and symptoms of bladder infection (cystitis) – frequency of passing urine, and burning and pain when passing urine. Sometimes a ureter (the tube through which urine passes from the kidney to the bladder) may become obstructed by the growth and may cause pain in the loin due to back-pressure on the kidney.

After losing blood in the urine for some time, anaemia may develop and symptoms of anaemia (pallor, tiredness, palpitations, etc.) may be noticed.

Investigations

The urine is examined for blood and may also be examined for cancer cells. Excretory urograms (IVP X-rays as described in Section 2) may show a filling defect or lump in the bladder. They may also show evidence of obstruction to a ureter if this is present.

A CT scan may reveal a lump in the bladder wall, but the ultimate investigation is with a cystoscope. The cystoscope (see Section 2) is passed into the bladder through the urethra (the tube for passage of urine from the bladder), usually under general anaesthesia, and the inside of the bladder is examined by the doctor. A small piece of any suspected cancer together with a small piece of adjacent bladder wall is taken as a biopsy for microscopic examination.

Types of bladder cancer (pathology)

There are various degrees of bladder tumours, ranging from a single benign cauliflower-like papilloma to an invasive, rigid, ulcerated and thickened cancer. Between these extremes there may be several papillomata (small warts or cauliflower-like growths), one or more of which may show signs of early malignancy, or there may be a malignant lump in the bladder wall. Bladder cancers tend to remain confined to the bladder wall for a long time before they spread. After a time, bladder cancers may involve the whole thickness of the bladder wall and even invade the rectum or other organs nearby in the pelvis. They may also spread to nearby lymph nodes, but do not commonly spread more widely.

Treatment

Small papillomata of the bladder are usually treated by burning them off with an instrument called an electro-cautery which is used through a cystoscope. The patient is cystoscoped regularly afterwards in case the tumour recurs.

For larger papillomas or early invasive cancers, treatment by radiotherapy or surgical excision or a combination of both radiotherapy and surgical excision may offer good prospects of cure.

For more advanced cancers it may be necessary to operate to remove the whole of the bladder (total cystectomy). A new type of bladder is then usually made by the surgeon from a part of the bowel.

When cure by surgery is not possible, palliative radiotherapy may give relief.

Chemotherapy has a limited place in the treatment of bladder cancer, although studies are being carried out in the hope of improving prospects of cure or worthwhile palliation with the use of newer agents and newer techniques of giving chemotherapy including by intra-arterial infusion.

KIDNEY CANCERS

Kidney cancers are not common, but there are three well recognised types. The Wilm's tumour or nephroblastoma occurs in children. In adults kidney cancers are either the adenocarcinoma (sometimes called hypernephroma or Grawitz tumour), or carcinoma of renal pelvis.

WILM'S TUMOUR (NEPHROBLASTOMA)

The Wilm's tumour usually is found in children of less than four years of age. It has even been found to be present at birth. Although in most cases only one kidney is affected, occasionally there is a cancer in both kidneys. This cancer is most commonly found as a lump in the loin of an infant. It may cause the child to be in general poor health with a fever, anaemia, or sometimes there may be blood in the urine. It may spread to nearby lymph nodes or into the large veins. From these veins cancer cells may be carried by the blood to the lungs, where secondary growths may develop.

ADENOCARCINOMA (GRAWITZ TUMOUR OR HYPERNEPHROMA)

This is the most common type of kidney cancer and is usually seen in adults of middle age or older age. The first symptom is usually the passage of blood in the urine, most often not associated with pain. (Passing of blood in the urine with pain in the loin is more likely to be caused by a kidney stone.) There may be a fever, or a lump may be felt in the loin, or sometimes there is local pain. This cancer may spread into nearby lymph nodes but commonly grows into the large renal vein (the vein taking blood from the kidney) and may spread by the bloodstream into the lungs, liver or bones. Sometimes the first evidence of this cancer is the presence of secondary cancers in a lung or in one or more bones.

CARCINOMA OF THE RENAL PELVIS

This cancer is rather like cancer of the bladder and behaves in a similar manner. The first sign is usually blood in the urine. This cancer sometimes develops as a reaction from a stone present in the kidney for a long time.

Investigations

X-rays of the abdomen may show an enlarged kidney. Excretory urograms (IVP), CT scans, ultrasound, and arteriography (see Section 2) are all useful investigations to help diagnose a tumour in a kidney and to help determine whether a kidney lump is solid and likely to be cancer, or a fluid-filled cyst and probably not malignant.

Other investigations include examination of the urine for blood or malignant cells and X-rays of lungs for evidence of secondary cancer. If there is evidence of swelling or painful areas in bones, these will be X-rayed and bone scans may be arranged to look for evidence of secondary bone cancers.

Treatment

Cancer of a kidney is best treated by surgical operation to remove the kidney (nephrectomy).

For Wilm's tumour (nephroblastoma) in children, results are much better if radiotherapy and chemotherapy are used in combination with surgical removal of the kidney.

For adenocarcinoma surgical treatment (removal of the kidney) is the only likely cure for a patient. Radiotherapy and chemotherapy may be used as palliative treatment in advanced cases, but results have been disappointing. Sometimes these cancers will show a temporary response to male or female hormones. Adenocarcinoma of the kidney is one cancer that sometimes spreads to a lung as one single secondary lump and this can sometimes be cured by an operation removing the part of the lung containing the single secondary lump.

For cancer of the renal pelvis, best results are achieved if the kidney is removed together with the whole of the ureter and a small part of the bladder as small seedlings of this cancer sometimes grow in the ureter between the kidney and the bladder.

Cancers of the brain

Although most brain cancers occur in people over the age of 45 years with a peak incidence between 60 and 70 years, the brain is also one of the more common sites for primary cancer in children and young adults.

There are two groups of cells in the brain that may form tumours. The glial cells (or true brain cells) from which most of the malignant tumours (cancers) develop, and the non-glial cells or supporting cells (such as cells of the meninges covering the brain or cells of the sheaths surrounding nerves) from which develop the majority of non-malignant (benign) tumours.

Cancers that arise from true brain cells or glial cells are called gliomas. There are a number of different types of gliomas, which range from the more slowly growing types called astrocytoma or oligodendroglioma to more rapidly and highly malignant types called medulloblastoma or glioblastoma multiforme. These different types of glioma tend to occur in different parts of the brain in children and adults. They also have other differences: the medulloblastomas are usually highly radio-sensitive and are sometimes cured by radiotherapy, but other types are less radio-sensitive if at all.

Symptoms and signs

Brain cancers tend to cause two types of clinical features:
- general features due to generalised pressure on the brain
- focal or local features due to pressure or interference by the tumour on parts of the brain or nerves near the tumour.

The common **general features** of cancer in the brain are due to pressure on and swelling of the brain as a whole. This causes headache, nausea, vomiting and disturbances of vision due to papilloedema (swelling of the optic nerve at the back of the

146

eye). Other features may be listlessness, tiredness and personality change. The sufferer may progressively withdraw from social contacts and gradually become confused, stuporous and may lapse into coma. In young children the increased pressure may cause the head to enlarge and hydrocephalus (so-called 'water on the brain') may develop.

It should be noted that in children, convulsions or fitting are most often caused by a fever or other less serious problem. Fitting alone is rarely caused by cancer in children. In an adult, however, with no previous history of epilepsy, injury or fitting from another known cause, the sudden onset of a fitting attack may be the first sign of a brain tumour.

Focal features are due to interference of function of a local region of brain. These features will depend upon the site of the tumour. In one place it may be interference with speech, in another it may be loss of movement of an arm or leg, in another place it may be loss of feeling or sensation of a part of the body. Tumours in other places may cause local twitching or focal fitting with different sensations such as sensation of smell or visual hallucinations like the flickering of lights. In other places there may be disorders of balance, or clumsy movement or interference with cranial nerves (the nerves that leave the brain) such as the optic nerves for vision, the nerves that move the eyeball or the facial nerves that move the muscles of the side of the face.

Investigations

The CT scan and MRI scan have revolutionised investigations for brain tumours. Before these scans were invented cerebral arteriography (X-rays of arteries supplying the brain), radio-isotope scans, and air encephalograms (see Section 2) were used almost routinely, together with a number of other investigations such as the EEG (electroencephalogram), which records brainwave activity. Nowadays, however, the CT scan (or the MRI scan) usually supplies most of the information of other investigations and even more precisely. Angiography may still give added information particularly concerning the vascularity of a tumour.

Treatment

Most benign cerebral tumours can be cured by surgical removal, but malignant tumours (brain cancers) are not often curable. For this reason, it is vital to determine – usually at operation – whether a tumour in the brain is benign or malignant (cancer). If malignant, it is also important to determine the type of malignancy, as the outlook for some is better than others and some (such as medulloblastomas) may be curable.

Although most are not curable, most patients with brain cancer can be given considerable relief of symptoms by a number of means. First, certain drugs (corticosteroids) can be used to reduce pressure on the brain and so relieve headaches and other pressure symptoms. Then surgical operation can be carried out to remove most of the cancer, giving further and more prolonged relief of symptoms. Following surgery the use of radiotherapy alone will usually further improve the immediate outlook.

Recent studies have shown that the use of post-operative chemotherapy with radiotherapy has given added benefit and some apparent cures have been reported, particularly in the case of medulloblastomas.

The leukaemias and lymphomas

THE LEUKAEMIAS

Leukaemia is a malignant growth or cancer of blood-forming cells. Leukaemias are of two main kinds according to the kind of blood-forming cell that has become malignant. These are called lymphatic leukaemia and myeloid leukaemia.

In lymphatic leukaemia the cells that have become malignant

are the bone marrow cells that normally make the white blood cells called lymphocytes. Lymph nodes and lymphoid tissue are usually involved and become enlarged. In myeloid leukaemia the cells that have become malignant are cells in the bone marrow which normally make the other types of white blood cells (e.g. polymorphs). The spleen usually becomes involved and enlarged.

Leukaemias may be acute or chronic according to whether the disease would tend to run a rapid and rapidly fatal course (acute leukaemia) or whether the disease would progress more slowly (chronic leukaemia). Thus there are four main types of leukaemia:

- acute lymphatic leukaemia (ALL)
- acute myeloid (or non-lymphatic) leukaemia (AML or ANLL)
- chronic lymphatic leukaemia (CLL)
- chronic myeloid (or non-lymphatic) leukaemia (CML or CNLL).

It is important to distinguish between the major types of leukaemia, as they tend to run different courses and respond differently to different drugs.

Leukaemia occurs throughout the world, but the incidence varies in different countries and in different races. All types of leukaemia are slightly more common in males. The Scandinavian countries and Israel have the highest incidence of leukaemia, and the lowest incidence is in Chile and Japan. In the USA the highest incidence is in Jews and the lowest is in Black Americans.

The overall incidence of acute lymphatic and acute myeloid leukaemia is about equal but there is a distinct age difference. Acute leukaemia accounts for about half of all cancers in children and acute lymphatic leukaemia is the most common of all cancers in young children, with a peak incidence of between two and four years. The incidence of acute myeloid leukaemia increases with age.

The causes of leukaemia are not known, although some pre-disposing factors are recognised. The myeloid leukaemias have been linked with ionising radiation and there is evidence that exposure of a foetus to X-rays during its mother's pregnancy is associated with a slightly increased risk of leukaemia developing later in childhood. However, there is no evidence that the normal use of diagnostic X-rays in adults is associated with leukaemia.

Excessive exposure to some chemical agents such as benzene is associated with a slightly increased risk of leukaemia. Acute myeloid leukaemia will also occasionally develop in patients who have had some other form of cancer including Hodgkin's lymphoma, or cancer of the ovary.

The use of anti-cancer cytotoxic drugs and especially the use of these drugs with radiotherapy also slightly increases the risk of later development of leukaemia.

Familial leukaemia is rare, although some families with multiple cases of leukaemia have been reported. In general, siblings of a child with leukaemia have only a slightly higher risk of developing leukaemia, although if one identical twin develops acute leukaemia the other twin has about a 20% chance of developing the disease.

People with Down's syndrome have a 20 times greater risk of developing acute leukaemia than normal people. Mothers of advancing age not only have an increased risk of producing children with Down's syndrome but normal children of mothers of advancing age also have a slightly greater risk of developing acute leukaemia.

Viruses are known to cause leukaemia in some animal species but there is no evidence that viruses cause leukaemia in humans.

THE ACUTE LEUKAEMIAS
Symptoms and signs

Symptoms are due to replacement of normal blood-forming cells of bone marrow by malignant leukaemic cells and infiltration (invasion) of other tissues such as spleen, lymph nodes, tonsils and sometimes liver, kidneys, lungs and brain.

Fever, weakness, anorexia (loss of appetite), pallor, and infection are common. Infection is especially common in the region of the tonsils or anus and the lungs may also become infected, causing pneumonia. There may be pain in bones or joints.

Lymph nodes, tonsils and spleen are commonly enlarged. Sometimes the liver and kidneys are enlarged.

There may be signs of bleeding from any site especially from the gums, the digestive tract or anus. Bleeding in the brain or from the lungs may also occur. Thromboses (clots) may also develop in veins.

Meningitis due to leukaemic cell spread into the meninges (the membranes covering the brain) frequently occurs in patients with acute lymphatic leukaemia unless prevented by radiotherapy or chemotherapy.

Investigations

The diagnosis can only be made after careful examination of blood and bone marrow. Blood is taken by a needle from a vein in the arm and bone marrow is usually taken with a small instrument that is used to puncture a bone of the pelvis (the iliac crest). Bone puncture is painful so is done under anaesthesia. A pathologist then examines the blood and bone marrow for leukaemic cells and for other features of leukaemia. These may include anaemia (with a reduction in numbers of red blood cells), reduction in number of normal white blood cells, and reduction in the number of platelets (the particles that help blood clotting).

Patients with acute myeloid leukaemia are usually found to have abnormalities of chromosomes. There may also be changes in blood chemistry such as increased uric acid (which may be associated with features of gout).

Treatment

Encouraging progress has been made in recent years in treatment of the acute leukaemias.

The best opportunity to achieve the maximum cure of leukaemia is when the disease is first diagnosed. Cells that remain after the first treatment tend to develop resistance to drugs. It is therefore important that patients with acute leukaemia should immediately be referred for specialist care so that the most effective treatment can be given under expert supervision from the beginning.

Chemotherapy using cytotoxic drugs and cortisone forms the basis of modern treatment. Combinations of effective cytotoxic drugs have produced best results.

With the best current treatment methods, over 90% of children and about 80% of adults with acute lymphatic leukaemia now achieve complete remission (that is, the disease apparently disappears and the patient feels and looks well again).

Anti-cancer drugs do not pass in high concentration into the brain. Because after a time most acute lymphatic leukaemic patients will develop the disease in the brain, injections of cytotoxic drugs are given into the meningeal space around the brain and the brain is also treated by radiotherapy. In the case of acute myeloid leukaemia, brain involvement does not occur so often, but this treatment is also given immediately there is any sign that there may be brain or central nervous system involvement.

With acute myeloid leukaemia, good results of chemotherapy have not been as reliable as with acute lymphatic leukaemia. Recently, in attempts to further improve results, bone marrow transplantation has been used effectively, especially in younger people (aged under 40 years). In marrow transplantation the leukaemic cells are destroyed by big doses of chemotherapy and radiotherapy (total body irradiation). This is a dangerous procedure and is only carried out in highly expert departments. The patient is then given injections of bone marrow taken from a matched donor (that is, a donor with similar body cells unlikely to cause a rejection reaction). The best donor is usually a parent or a sibling. Bone marrow transplantation involves a number of risks and problems and can only be carried out by appropriately trained experts in especially equipped hospitals, but results have been most encouraging in this otherwise fatal illness. A further encouraging development is quite new at the time of writing. When a good matching bone marrow donor is not available, umbilical cord blood has been used as an alternative with good results in children and in some small adults.

In recent years, treatment with immunotherapy has been further investigated. Although major success has not as yet been achieved there have been some interesting results which give hope for better treatments becoming available in the future.

During the acute illness there may be special problems of anaemia, lowered resistance to infection, bleeding or even clotting. These may require blood transfusion or platelet transfusion. Aspirin should be strictly avoided as it interferes with blood clotting.

CHRONIC MYELOID (GRANULOCYTIC) LEUKAEMIA

Chronic myeloid leukaemia can occur at any age, but its highest incidence is between the ages of 30 and 50 years. Although there is no known cause in most cases, it was found that in Japan five to eight years after the atomic bomb explosions there was an increase in both acute and chronic myeloid leukaemia.

In chronic myeloid leukaemia there is a great increase in the number of white cells in the blood. This is associated with a big increase in the number of cells in bone marrow. There may also be a considerable increase in the numbers of blood platelets (the particles in blood responsible for clotting).

Symptoms and signs

One of the more common symptoms is pain in the left upper abdomen due to an enlarged spleen. The spleen is usually easily felt in patients with this disease (a normal spleen cannot be felt with examining fingers). There may also be features of anaemia, tiredness, weight loss or fever. Sometimes, abnormal bruising, bleeding or clotting problems may be the first evidence of the disease.

Investigations

Blood count and bone marrow biopsy will usually establish the diagnosis.

Treatment

There are two phases of chronic myeloid leukaemia. The chronic phase is the least dangerous and with modern treatment may last for many months or years before the dangerous acute phase takes over.

During the chronic phase the disease can usually be kept under good control with cytotoxic chemotherapy. The drug most commonly used with good effect is busulphan, although other drugs may also give good disease control. With this treatment the blood count may return to normal and the spleen may be reduced considerably in size.

However, if the spleen remains large and causes pain or other problems due to its large size and over-activity it may sometimes be necessary to have the spleen removed by a surgeon.

Sooner or later, a more acute and more dangerous episode of this disease will develop resembling acute myeloid leukaemia. This phase of the disease is more difficult to control. Sometimes other cytotoxic chemotherapy with cortisone might give control for a period. Experimental studies are also being made to control this acute phase of the disease with intensive radiotherapy and bone marrow transplantation but a number of problems still need to be overcome. Control of the acute phase of this disease remains a difficult problem.

CHRONIC LYMPHATIC (LYMPHOCYTIC) LEUKAEMIA

Chronic lymphatic leukaemia tends to occur in older people of an average of about 60 years of age. In this disease there is an overproduction of mature and relatively normal looking lymphocytes with increased numbers of lymphocytes in the blood. (Lymphocytes are one of the main types of white cells in the blood. They are in high concentration in lymph nodes and some other tissues.)

Symptoms and signs

The most obvious feature is lymph node enlargement. Enlarged lymph nodes may be felt as lumps in the sides of the neck, in the armpits (axillae) or groins. Enlarged lymph nodes in the abdomen are more difficult to feel but enlarged lymph nodes in the chest may be detected on a chest X-ray. The spleen and sometimes the liver may also be enlarged. The normal bone marrow may be replaced by malignant lymphocytes and the patient may become anaemic (deficient in red cells) and deficient in the circulating clotting particles called platelets. This may lead to bleeding and clotting problems. Due to the replacement of normal white cells by abnormal white cells the patient has decreased ability to combat infection and may also have immunologic abnormalities.

Investigations

Blood count, bone marrow biopsy and special tests of immune function will establish the diagnosis.

Treatment

Chronic lymphatic leukaemia is usually a very slowly progressive disease and many patients may not need treatment for months or years. There is no evidence that the disease can be cured by early treatment and treatment is usually reserved for episodes of the disease that are causing the patient to feel ill or causing other problems.

Large and conspicuous lymph nodes and a large spleen can be reduced by radiotherapy. If the patient's general health is poor, treatment with anti-cancer cytotoxic drugs, often with cortisone, will usually cause reduction of enlarged lymph nodes and spleen, improve the bone marrow and will make the patient feel better. Two cytotoxic anti-cancer drugs are commonly used – chlorambucil and cyclophosphamide. Both are given by mouth.

Unlike chronic myeloid leukaemia, chronic lymphatic leukaemia does not degenerate into an acute type of leukaemia. However, it may occasionally change into a lymphoma-like disease as described below.

THE LYMPHOMAS

The lymphomas are a group of malignant diseases (cancers) of the body tissues that constitute the body defence system known as the reticulo-endothelial or immune system. That is, the lymphomas arise in lymph nodes or in lymphoid tissue elsewhere as in the tonsils, the spleen, the wall of stomach or bowel, the liver, lung, kidneys or skin.

There are two main types of lymphoma: Hodgkin's lymphoma

(or Hodgkin's disease) and the so-called non-Hodgkin's lymphomas.

About half the cases of lymphoma are Hodgkin's lymphoma, which predominantly originates in lymph nodes. The non-Hodgkin's lymphomas develop almost as commonly in lymphoid tissue in other organs as much as they do in lymph nodes.

Lymphomas are the seventh most common cause of death from cancer in the USA and commonly occur in young people. The average age is about 30 years for Hodgkin's lymphoma and a little over 40 years for non-Hodgkin's lymphoma.

The causes of most lymphomas are not known. Viruses are known to be a cause of lymphomas in some animals but, with one exception, viruses have not been found to be a significant cause of lymphoma in humans. A lymphoma called Burkitt's lymphoma, which is uncommon in most countries but is common in children in tropical Africa, has been found to be associated with infection by a virus called the Epstein-Barr virus. This same virus causes glandular fever and it has been found that in Western societies people who have suffered from glandular fever have a slightly increased risk of developing a lymphoma later in life. On the other hand, doctors and nurses who specialise in caring for people with lymphoma have not been found to have any increased risk of developing the disease.

It is well recognised that people with a deficiency of their immune systems, especially AIDS patients, but also others such as people who have had a kidney transplant and are given drugs to suppress the rejection of the transplanted kidney, have an increased risk of developing a lymphoma. There is also a slightly increased tendency to develop lymphomas in some families, but this may be due to an hereditary tendency towards immune deficiency.

HODGKIN'S DISEASE (HODGKIN'S LYMPHOMA)
Symptoms and signs

The most common sign, especially in young people, is of enlarged lymph nodes, usually in one or other side of the neck. The nodes are rubbery and movable and usually feel distinctly different to the hard enlarged nodes that may result from secondary spread from other cancers.

Sometimes, other symptoms are present – malaise (a general feeling of ill health), fever or weight loss. Occasionally, pain in swollen lymph nodes following drinking alcohol is a feature.

The disease usually progresses from the site of origin (most commonly lymph nodes in the neck) to other lymph nodes nearby – then to lymph nodes in the chest or abdomen – to the spleen – and eventually to the liver and bone marrow. The earlier the disease is detected before it has spread widely the greater the likelihood of cure by modern treatment.

Investigations

In order to decide on the best treatment for a patient it is important to find out as accurately as possible which lymph nodes and which organs are involved with this form of cancer. If this disease is suspected the doctor performs a thorough examination of the patient, including all lymph node areas, spleen, liver and chest. X-rays are taken of the lungs especially to look for enlarged lymph nodes in the chest (mediastinal lymph nodes).

The doctor then makes sure of the diagnosis by having the most obvious and easily removed lymph node excised by a surgeon to have it examined under a microscope. Thus a diagnosis can be made. In fact, any patient who has a lymph node greater than 1.5 cm in diameter remaining enlarged for more than a month or 6 weeks without an obvious cause should have that node removed and examined in case it is an early indication of a serious disease like Hodgkin's disease.

If a positive diagnosis of Hodgkin's disease is made, a number of other tests should be done. A blood count is arranged, as anaemia may develop and other features of Hodgkin's disease may also be found in the blood.

CT scans and ultrasound help in discovering if there are any enlarged lymph nodes in the abdomen as well as any enlargement of the liver or spleen.

Lymphoscintigrams and gallium isotope scans (see Section 2) may now be used to show abnormal or enlarged lymph nodes.

The value of PET scans in detecting affected tissues and in assessing response to treatment is presently under study.

A liver biopsy and bone narrow biopsy may indicate involvement of these tissues with disease.

Studies of kidney function may also indicate possible involvement of the kidneys.

Treatment

Some patients who had Hodgkin's disease a few years ago will remember that an operation was done by a surgeon to find out what organs and tissues in the abdomen were involved with Hodgkin's disease (a staging laparotomy). This operation is hardly ever needed nowadays because of the accuracy of CT scans, ultrasound, isotope scans, gallium scans and lympho-scintigram studies. These may even be replaced one day by PET scans, but not yet. PET scans are not widely available, and in any case it is still uncertain as to whether they will be as reliable and accurate as the combined information from the other tests (see Section 2).

Treatment of Hodgkin's disease is either by radiotherapy or by chemotherapy or both. Treatment must be given by experts experienced in treating this disease, as well delivered treatment can now improve greatly the outlook for this once lethal illness. It is now possible to cure most patients, especially those who do not have extensive disease.

In general, limited areas of disease are best treated by radiotherapy (a modern linear accelerator is the most appropriate equipment) but the exact doses, techniques of delivery and field of irradiation must be expertly arranged.

For widespread disease in which tissue other than just lymph nodes and spleen are involved, treatment is usually by chemotherapy – using appropriate combinations of cytotoxic drugs. Again, to achieve best results and to keep toxic side-effects (see Section 2) to a minimum, treatment should be given by experts who are familiar with the use of these drugs and experienced in treating lymphomas.

NON-HODGKIN'S LYMPHOMAS

Like Hodgkin's disease, this group of diseases begins in reticuloendothelial tissues (the immune body defence system) and may first be noticed in lymph nodes. However, the first indication of non-Hodgkin's lymphomas may be enlargement or lumps in the spleen, tonsils, or other organs such as stomach, bowel, lung, bone or skin.

Non-Hodgkin's lymphoma is not just one disease. There is a range of diseases of the reticulo-endothelial system grouped together and called the non-Hodgkin's lymphomas. The particular type of lymphoma depends upon the predominant type of malignant cell.

Investigations

Diagnosis is usually made by surgical removal of an enlarged lymph node or biopsy of a lump in another tissue with microscopic examination.

Non-Hodgkin's lymphomas tend to behave according to the

predominant type of malignant cell. As with Hodgkin's disease, staging operations are rarely needed. In the non-Hodgkin's lymphomas the disease tends to involve a number of tissues other than lymph nodes and the best form of treatment will depend upon the predominant type of malignant cell rather than the types of tissue involved. However, similar investigations as for Hodgkin's disease are usually required including full blood count, chest X-ray, CT scan, bone marrow biopsies, liver biopsy and lymphangiograms. PET scans may be of additional diagnostic help when more readily available in the future (see Section 2).

Treatment

Just as for Hodgkin's disease, treatment of the non-Hodgkin's lymphomas is by radiotherapy, chemotherapy or both. However, depending on the type of lymphoma, different plans of radiotherapy or different programs of chemotherapy are used. It is therefore essential that the patient be treated by a team of experts who can best determine the type and extent of disease and arrange the most appropriate plan of radiotherapy or chemotherapy or both.

In general, radiotherapy is best used for localised disease. With the non-Hodgkin's lymphomas, however, there is a considerable risk that the disease is present in more than one site or in more than one tissue and treatment by general body chemotherapy (systemic chemotherapy) is usually required. Sometimes in some types of lymphoma, the use of one cytotoxic agent only will achieve good results, though in general best results are achieved when a combination of two or more cytotoxic drugs is used.

Over recent years, results of treatment of most non-Hodgkin's lymphomas have improved significantly with modern treatment regimens. This is especially so in some specific types of lymphoma. For some younger patients even with advanced disease very high dose toxic treatment followed by a bone marrow transplant may be used with a good chance of success.

A new approach under study combines the techniques of genetic engineering with immunotherapy. Genetic engineering is used to modify antibody-producing cells in animals (mice) so that they produce antibodies against human malignant cells (non-Hodgkin's lymphoma) but not against normal human cells. Clinical application of this approach is currently under study, and encouraging tumour responses have been recorded, but as yet a number of problems remain to be solved, including the high cost of producing such antibodies in clinically effective quantities.

Soft tissue sarcomas

The soft tissues are those tissues that surround the bones of the body and include muscles, fat, fascia, nerves, tendons, blood vessels and lymphatic vessels. A malignant tumour of one of these tissues is, strictly speaking, not a cancer but a sarcoma. However, the term cancer is often used as a sarcoma is a malignancy in many ways similar to cancer.

The majority of soft tissue tumours are not malignant – it is only when they are malignant that the term sarcoma applies. Thus most tumours of fatty tissue are lipomas – it is only when one of these is malignant that it is called a liposarcoma. Similarly, most tumours of fibrous tissue are benign and are called fibromas, and most tumours of nerves are benign and are called neuromas. Most blood and lymph vessel tumours are benign and are called angiomas.

Thus sarcomas are classified according to the type of tissue from which they arise and the type of tissue they most resemble. A fibrosarcoma is therefore a malignant tumour or cancer of fibrous tissue; a liposarcoma is a malignant tumour or cancer of fatty tissue; a neurosarcoma is a malignant tumour or cancer of nerve tissue; a malignant fibrous histiocytoma (MFH) is a sarcoma of histiocytes (protective cells most often in soft tissues) and a synovial sarcoma is a malignant tumour of the synovial membrane that lines joints and tendon sheaths. A myosarcoma is a malignant tumour of muscle.

Myosarcomas may be further classified as rhabdomyo-sarcoma and leiomyosarcoma. A rhabdomyosarcoma is a malignant tumour of a voluntary muscle (that is, one of the muscles of the body over which we have control in moving arms, legs, abdomen, back, head and neck or the muscles used in breathing). A leiomyosarcoma is a malignant tumour of invol-untary muscle (that is, one of the muscles over which we have no conscious control) such as the muscle in the wall of the stomach or bowel, or the muscles in the wall of the uterus or the wall of large blood vessels.

An angiosarcoma is a malignant tumour of blood or lymph vessels. In the case of blood vessels it is called a haemangio-sarcoma or in the case of lymphatic vessels it is called lymphan-giosarcoma.

Soft tissue sarcomas occur in people of all ages from birth to old age but they are much less common than are true cancers. Soft tissue sarcomas make up only about 2% of malignant tumours.

In general, sarcomas have a tendency to recur locally after surgical excision and also to spread. While most cancers tend to spread via the lymph vessels to lymph nodes before they spread to lungs or other body organs, most sarcomas, on the other hand, have a greater tendency to spread via blood vessels to lungs rather than to lymph nodes.

CLASSIFICATION – PATHOLOGICAL TYPES
Fibrosarcoma

These tumours develop in fascia or fibrous tissue that covers and surrounds muscles, nerves and other tissues and is distributed widely throughout the body. Thus a fibrosarcoma may develop almost anywhere in the body, especially in a limb or in the tissues of the trunk. One very fibrous and slowly growing type of fibrosarcoma called a desmoid tumour has a tendency to grow into nearby tissues and to recur locally after surgical excision but rarely spreads to other organs. Other more cellular and less fibrous types have a greater tendency to spread.

Liposarcoma

These tumours develop from fatty tissue and may arise anywhere in the body where fat is present. They tend to vary from a low grade malignancy likely to recur locally after operations for their removal but unlikely to spread, to a high grade malignancy in which both local recurrence and secondary spread to lungs is common.

Rhabdomyosarcoma

This tumour presents as a swelling in voluntary muscle, especially in muscles in the limbs, and is the sarcoma most likely to spread to lymph nodes.

Leiomyosarcoma

This tumour may occur at any site where there is smooth muscle including the wall of the stomach or bowel or the uterus or the wall of large blood vessels.

Neurosarcoma

This tumour may develop on any nerve. Sometimes it is purely a tumour of nerve cells, and sometimes it is a mixture of fibrous tissue and nerve tissue and it may then be called a neuro-fibrosarcoma.

Malignant fibrous histiocytoma (MFH)

These tumours most commonly develop in muscles, fascia or fatty tissues in limbs. They are firm rounded tumours rather like liposarcomas or fibrosarcomas. If deep in muscle they may become quite large before they are noticed as they cause few symptoms until a lump is felt.

Angiosarcoma

These tumours may develop in relation to blood vessels or lymph vessels and develop as enlarging vascular masses (clumps containing partly formed blood vessels). They are softish tumours that may contain either blood or lymphatic fluid.

Synovial sarcoma (synoviosarcoma or malignant synovioma)

This tumour of synovial membrane is often a highly aggressive malignant tumour and occurs most commonly in limbs near joints or in association with the sheaths around muscle tendons.

Symptoms and signs

Sarcomas occasionally develop from previously benign tumours of a similar type. Thus occasionally a previously benign lipoma, for example, will begin to enlarge, showing evidence of a malignant liposarcoma. More often, however, these tumours arise as a local swelling from no apparent pre-existing abnormality. Usually the lump is not painful although sometimes there is some pain. Occasionally the swelling develops at a site of recent injury and the possibility of a sarcoma developing as a result of injury cannot be dismissed. It is more likely, however, that in most cases the injury drew attention to a lump which was already present.

Rarely, the first evidence of a soft tissue sarcoma is found in a chest X-ray showing as secondary lung cancer.

Investigations

The examining doctor will first ask about the lump, especially how long it has been present and if, when and how rapidly it started to enlarge. The lump is measured, the local draining lymph nodes and other lymph nodes will be examined and a chest X-ray and full blood count will be performed. CT scan, ultrasound and angiography (see Section 2) may also give more information about the tumour and sometimes MRI studies will help, but the final diagnosis will be made by taking a biopsy specimen of the lump for microscopic examination.

Whether further information of value can be learned from PET scans is presently being investigated.

Treatment

The standard treatment of soft tissue sarcoma is excision at a surgical operation. As the risk of local recurrence of sarcoma is high, the surgeon must remove a great deal of apparently normal tissue around the tumour to be as sure as possible that all of the malignant cells have been removed. Often in a limb, and especially for large tumours, amputation of the limb may be recommended as offering the best chance of cure.

Although these tumours are usually not particularly sensitive to radiotherapy, sometimes radiotherapy combined with local surgery may achieve better results than surgery alone.

Many of these tumours will respond to cytotoxic chemotherapy. Early medical experience with the use of chemotherapy to treat secondary sarcoma, especially in the lungs, achieved some regression with improved length of survival for some patients, but dramatic improvement in results has not been achieved. More recently, chemotherapy has also been used before operation to reduce the size, extent and vitality of the primary tumour before surgery. When the chemotherapy can be given by regional infusion into a supplying artery (as in the case of a sarcoma in a limb), encouraging results have been achieved. The chemotherapy is given first into the artery supplying blood to the sarcoma followed by its surgical resection. Results of this combined treatment have often avoided the need for amputation in patients in whom it would otherwise have been required. Such combined treatment should now be considered by experts experienced in these techniques before amputation is carried out.

Liposarcomas and malignant fibrous histiocytomas are the most common of the soft tissue sarcomas, and even when very large they usually respond well to regional chemotherapy given before surgery, making follow-up surgical removal possible and successful in most cases, without amputation.

With some sarcomas, the risk of secondary spread to lungs is considerable and there may be virtue in also giving a post-operative course of adjuvant chemotherapy (see Section 2) to reduce the risk of secondary lung cancer developing. Studies are being carried out to determine whether the outlook for patients with aggressive sarcoma can be further improved with this treatment.

Malignant tumours of bone and cartilage

OSTEOSARCOMA

A malignant tumour of bone-forming cells is called an osteosarcoma. This is an uncommon but highly malignant form of cancer and tends to affect children and young adults, with the highest incidence between 10 and 25 years of age. The cause of osteosarcoma in young people is not known, although it does occur most often in the growing parts of bone near the bone ends while the patient is still growing,

A rare and incurable osteosarcoma sometimes develops in old people, but these people almost always have a longstanding bone disease called osteitis deformans or Paget's disease of bone.

Symptoms and signs

Osteosarcoma usually first develops as a painful lump near the end of a bone. There may be an obvious swelling occasionally with overlying redness and sometimes a fever. The swelling may be tender and may at first look like an acute infection in bone. This sarcoma tends to spread to the lungs early in its course so that best results are achieved if it is diagnosed and treated very early before secondary spread to the lungs has taken place.

Investigations

Bone X-rays often show a typical appearance of the disease in which a diagnosis of osteosarcoma can be made. More precise information can be learned from CT studies or MRI studies. PET scans if available may give even further information about the tumour. However, the ultimate deciding test is a bone biopsy in which a small piece of the tumour is taken for microscopic examination. Chest X-rays will also be taken to look for evidence of spread to the lungs.

Treatment

Twenty-five years ago, osteosarcoma could rarely be cured. Treatment was by early amputation of an affected limb, sometimes in combination with radiotherapy, but death usually resulted due to development of secondary cancer in the lungs.

The outlook has been greatly improved with modern chemotherapy. Nowadays cytotoxic drugs are given as adjuvant chemotherapy (see Section 2) from the time of diagnosis. Amputation has usually been used to eradicate the primary sarcoma and the chemotherapy is used to eradicate any microscopic secondary cancers in the lungs before they develop into larger incurable cancers. From almost no cures previously the cure rate was improved to about 50% but in virtually all cured patients a limb was amputated.

In some clinics the use of chemotherapy is now taken even further. Rather than amputation of the limb, regional chemotherapy is first given to the limb by infusing cytotoxic drugs into the artery supplying the limb with blood. This treatment is then followed by surgery to remove the tissues containing the original tumour without amputating the limb. The section of bone that contained the tumour must be removed and replaced by an artificial prosthesis made of metal or plastic material. This operation must be carried out by a highly skilled and experienced orthopaedic surgeon. If there is any doubt about any malignant cells still being present radiotherapy might also be given after the surgery. Adjuvant chemotherapy is thereafter given for some months to destroy any undetected microscopic collections of cancer cells in the lungs or other parts of the body. This combined treatment is very effective in curing more than half of the patients with osteosarcoma and in 80% of these cases the cure is achieved without amputating a limb.

In some clinics the pre-operative chemotherapy is not given into the artery supplying the limb but is given systemically (into a vein). This is an easier method of giving chemotherapy and results of treatment are possibly as good as with intra-arterial chemotherapy for this tumour.

OSTEOCLASTOMA (CENTRAL GIANT CELL TUMOUR OF BONE)

This tumour occurs most commonly in the ends of long bones of middle-aged adults. It is a tumour of low-grade malignancy in that it does not often spread to other organs or tissues, but tends to develop locally, and commonly recurs locally after attempts at removal.

Symptoms and signs

The first evidence of this tumour is usually swelling, often with pain. It may be first noticed due to a fracture of the weakened bone.

Investigations

X-rays, CT or MRI will usually show a typical appearance of this tumour but diagnosis is established by the surgeon taking a biopsy specimen and having it examined by a pathologist under the microscope.

Treatment

If possible, the tumour is removed surgically. If inadequately removed, radiotherapy may be given post-operatively.

A recurrent tumour tends to be more malignant and treatment by amputation may be required.

EWING'S TUMOUR

This is an uncommon malignant tumour that occurs most often in the shafts of long bones of adolescents and young adults. Although it occurs in bones, it is not truly a tumour of bone cells but is a tumour of connective tissue in bone.

Symptoms and signs

Pain, swelling, fever and anaemia are common features of Ewing's tumour, so much so that a diagnosis of infection (osteomyelitis) may be thought to be present. Sometimes lesions are present in more than one bone.

Investigations

X-rays of the bone often show a laminated 'onion peel' appearance that is typical of Ewing's tumour. Further useful information may be gained from CT or MRI studies or from isotope scans. Biopsy and microscopic examination will establish the diagnosis.

This is a tumour where, if available, PET scans may be especially helpful to detect any focus of tumour in bones at other sites and to see evidence of a response to chemotherapy and radiotherapy treatment.

Treatment

Standard treatment by surgery (usually amputation) has rarely cured this highly malignant tumour.

With modern treatment using chemotherapy, radiotherapy and possibly local surgical excision significantly better results are now being achieved.

MULTIPLE MYELOMA

This tumour also occurs in bone but is not truly a tumour of bone. It is in fact a tumour of a type of blood-forming cell in bone, but presents as a lump or lumps in one or more bones. Usually there are many lumps in a number of bones, although occasionally a single lump only is present.

Multiple myeloma most often affects adults over 40 or 50 years. It causes local pain and swelling in affected bones and there may be a fracture of a bone.

Investigations

X-rays may show typical 'punched out' areas in bones. A blood count is taken, as the patients are usually found to have anaemia. Other changes in the blood proteins may confirm the diagnosis of this disease.

The urine is also examined for a particular type of protein (Bence-Jones protein) which, if present, indicates a diagnosis of multiple myeloma.

Treatment

As this tumour is usually widespread, it cannot be eradicated by surgery. Treatment by chemotherapy with local radiotherapy to painful lumps offers the best relief of symptoms and some-times long-term control is achieved. Treatment of anaemia may require blood transfusion.

CHONDROSARCOMA

Chondrosarcoma is a malignant tumour of cartilage and most often affects middle-aged adults. This tumour may develop on any bone, especially at the ends of long bones or in bones of the pelvis. It is usually first noticed as a slowly growing painful lump on a bone, often near a large joint.

Investigations

X-rays will often show typical appearance of a chondrosarcoma, but biopsy will establish the diagnosis. CT or MRI studies will help show the exact position, nature and extent of the tumour.

Treatment

If possible, radical surgical excision of the tumour with adja-cent bone is carried out – this may require amputation of a limb. These sarcomas are not sensitive to radiotherapy or to chemotherapy, but as they are slow growing and usually do not spread until late in the disease, treatment by radical surgery usually results in cure.

Secondary or metastatic cancer

A secondary or metastatic cancer is a cancer that is growing in an organ or tissue some distance away from the tissue or organ in which it originated. The most important differences between benign tumours and malignant tumours are that benign tumours tend to grow very slowly and remain localised to the tissue in which they arise, whereas malignant tumours (cancers) tend to grow more rapidly, to grow into surrounding structures and damage them, and to spread into tissues or organs away from the original or primary site of development. To spread to distant sites, the malignant cells usually grow into blood vessels or lymph vessels and clumps of cells break off and are carried by the bloodstream or the lymphatic vessels to a distant organ or tissue or to lymph nodes where they may grow as secondary tumours. The spreading cancer cells can be seen as 'seeds' being transported along blood or lymph vessels to a new 'soil' where they may take root and grow. Malignant cells may also sometimes spread along nerve sheaths, or across body cavities such as the abdominal cavity or a pleural cavity in the chest.

The most common site for secondary spread of cancers is via lymph vessels into lymph nodes. First they grow in lymph nodes near the original cancer and then spread into lymph nodes further away. The next most common sites are the lungs or the liver, by spread through the bloodstream.

Other common sites of secondary spread are to bones, the brain, under the skin, or to the ovaries. No tissue, including the adrenal glands and the kidneys, is exempt from developing a secondary cancer. However, some organs and tissues tend to have a relatively low incidence of secondary growth of most cancers for no obvious reason. These include the spleen and muscles.

The likelihood of a tumour spreading to a particular site depends very much on the type of tumour and its place of origin. Stomach, pancreas and bowel cancers, for example, tend to spread first to abdominal lymph nodes and to the liver. Breast cancer tends to spread to nearby lymph nodes, to the liver, lungs and bone. Prostate cancer tends to spread to bone. Skin cancer and cancers in the mouth and throat tend to spread to nearby lymph nodes; the exception is BCC, which rarely spreads anywhere other than into surrounding tissues. Melanoma, on the other hand, tends to spread early not only to lymph nodes but to almost any other organ or tissue in the body.

Sarcomas do not usually spread to lymph nodes first but are more likely to first spread via the bloodstream to the lungs.

More detail about the spread of each different type of cancer has been discussed under its appropriate heading earlier in this section. The treatment of secondary cancer depends on the type and site of origin of the particular tumour; it has similarly been discussed under the individual headings in this section.

Where do we go from here?

4

The future for cancer patients is a mixture of hope and caution. Certainly there is much that can be done by skilled application of present knowledge. There is also a great deal of expectation of improvements in prevention, diagnosis and care in the future.

However, just as there will be great advances in prevention and management of cancer in the future, so too will there be new challenges. The condition AIDS (acquired immune deficiency syndrome) is one such example: it is a new health problem unknown 20 years ago. Affected people have increased susceptibility to infections and to malignant tumour development. As yet no cure is in sight. Those who have had organ transplants and are dependent on immunosuppressive drugs to prevent rejection of the organ also have an increased risk of developing cancer. This is a relatively new problem, unknown 40 years ago. The sexual revolution has exposed young women to an increased risk of cancer of the cervix. It is not known what potential other modern drugs, especially the illegal drugs, might have to increase the risk of cancer: it took many years before the dangers of tobacco smoking became obvious. Studies suggest that for long-term smokers of marijuana, the risk of cancer is similar to that for tobacco smokers.

Prevention

The most obvious way to reduce the risk of cancer is to avoid smoking. This has been known for some years, but human nature being what it is, this precaution has been widely disregarded. As long as there are large profits to be made from the sale of tobacco products there will be resistance to the introduction of statutory measures aimed at reducing smoking.

Another useful active measure is to encourage fair-skinned people to take greater protection against exposure to the sun.

More attention can be paid to removal of pre-malignant conditions like hyperkeratoses, leukoplakia, stomach and bowel polyps and papillomas and to the prevention of such infections as hepatitis and HIV.

Diet and changes in lifestyle

Changes in lifestyle include a reduction of animal fats and artificial additives and other contaminants in the diet and a greater intake of fibre, fresh fruits and vegetables, nuts and protective legumes. Moderation in the use of alcohol should be encouraged. There will continue to be advances based on epidemiological information and a better understanding of the protective qualities of high fibre diets including the apparent protective qualities of other agents such as the naturally occurring hormones (the phytoestrogens) present in soy and other plant foods.

Open-mindedness towards 'alternative' and naturopathic practices

More might be learned from alternative medicine and naturo-pathic practices as well as traditional practices from ancient and undeveloped communities. Several effective anti-cancer drugs are extracted from plants used in other cultures, and it is likely that other such anti-cancer agents will be discovered among plants being used in other cultures or by alternative practices. However, care must be taken to properly analyse such practices and not allow wishful thinking, emotion or fashion to cloud scientific and clinical judgment.

Improved environmental and industrial laws and practices

Reduction of atmospheric pollutants, vigilant observation of pro-tective industrial laws and protection against radioactive sources are also important preventive factors.

Improved cancer screening

Another measure of increasing importance is regular screening of people at special risk for certain types of cancer so that any early lesions can be detected and treated before an advanced cancer develops. At present this seems to be the most appropriate way to detect early breast cancer, skin cancers including melanoma, cancer of the cervix, cancer of the stomach (in some communi-ties) and large bowel cancer.

It is anticipated that simpler and more accurate screening measures will be available in the future. These may include simple blood screening tests for cancer antibodies or other tumour markers to indicate the presence of early cancer before symptoms have developed and at a more curable stage.

Early detection and treatment – improved diagnostic techniques

Improved diagnostic measures will also allow more accurate diagnosis at an earlier stage. Already improvements in CT scanning and other organ imaging techniques have made considerable advances and further advances are assured. Magnetic resonance imaging (MRI) has added to these improved diagnostic and imaging methods. It is anticipated that the newer method of organ imaging, PET (positron emission tomography), may make an even greater impact within a few years because of the additional information it gives about the activity, composition and survival of tumour cells and its capacity to detect secondary cells at an earlier stage than has been possible in the past.

Fine needle aspiration cytology, frozen section techniques and other improved pathology techniques have allowed major progress in detecting and establishing the nature of tumours. Improvements in the ability to examine body cavities with the use of flexible fibrescopes have allowed considerable progress in detecting and assessing early cancers in recent years. These instruments and their applications will undoubtedly continue to be improved.

Improved agents and more effective use of chemotherapy

Improved treatment with more effective and more specific anti-cancer drugs is progressing as is knowledge of how best to use such drugs in combinations and treatment schedules to achieve greater anti-tumour effects with a reduced risk of toxicity and unwanted side-effects. New and more effective anti-cancer agents such as the new plant extracts known as the *Taxanes* are adding to the range of available anti-cancer drugs. The use of many drugs is being made safer and more effective with the increasing availability of agents that protect bone marrow and other body tissues.

Solving many of the problems of bone marrow transplantation has also allowed stronger and more effective anti-cancer treatment to be given with improved safety. It is anticipated that heavy dose chemotherapy with bone marrow transplantation will be used effectively to treat patients with many more advanced cancers than the limited number of tumour types (mostly lymphomas and leukaemias) for which this treatment is presently used with relative safety. There is already evidence that these techniques may be effective in treating some women with advanced widespread breast cancers. Such treatment schedules may be further expanded by recent information about the value of foetal blood from the umbilical cord of newborn babies as an alternative source of bone marrow-like cells. It is likely that foetal blood banks will be developed for such treatment programs in the future.

New laboratory testing methods will also provide information as to which treatment methods and which anti-cancer agents are likely to be of greatest benefit in treating each cancer.

Improvements in radiotherapy

Treatment by radiotherapy is also being constantly improved with different types of radio-emission and different treatment schedules integrated with anti-cancer drugs or hormones for more effective treatment. Methods are being developed to more directly target tumour cells for irradiation and so reduce risk of damage to normal cells.

More effective use of chemotherapy and radiotherapy integrated with surgery

Although a greater use of less invasive surgery with improved flexible scopes is likely, it seems otherwise that operative surgical measures for cancer will not advance greatly over present practice. Possible exceptions might be a greater use of organ replacement and regional tissue perfusion techniques. However, there may be an increasing role for better planned, integrated treatment schedules in which chemotherapy, radiotherapy and surgical methods are used more effectively in combination from the outset to improve treatment of advanced cancers. Surgical measures and radiological catheter techniques to distribute anti-cancer agents more selectively and in greater concentration to the region of a tumour are presently undergoing further studies. It is anticipated that in the future, with PET scan imaging, treatment will be directed even more selectively to parts of the body where it is needed.

Heat therapy and cryosurgery

Another treatment possibility, as yet not well exploited, involves the known increased susceptibility of cancer cells to heat. Studies of the application of heat to selectively eradicate tumour cells, possibly in combination with anti-cancer drugs, may produce improved treatment techniques for certain types of cancer in the future. At the same time, the application of extreme cold to cancer cells (cryosurgery) is being further developed, especially as a technique to cure secondary cancers in the liver.

Immunotherapy

Perhaps the greatest hope for the future is in the field of immunotherapy. Cancers are often thought to be caused by a deficiency in the body's immune defence system. Whereas abnormal cells are usually recognised and eradicated by the body's immune defences, in the cancer patient the abnormal cells have continued to survive and multiply. There is a great deal of supportive evidence for this 'immune surveillance theory', but one form of evidence is that there have been very occasional reports of an advanced and aggressive type of cancer which suddenly and spontaneously disappeared without trace for no apparent reason. This suggests that somehow the body's natural defence mechanisms may have taken charge again.

A great deal of work has been carried out in leading hospitals, cancer centres and other institutions in the search for greater knowledge of immunological defence mechanisms. There is hope that specific immunological tumour markers will reveal the presence of certain cancers very early and before they can otherwise be clinically detected. There is hope that tumour antibodies may not only reveal early evidence of cancer, but may be used in treatment, either in a direct attack on, or by carrying specific cytotoxic chemical agents to, the cancer cells. There is hope that a more reliable means of stimulating the immune defence system will emerge from these studies. Preparations of monoclinal antibodies (antibodies active against the specific type of cancer cell only) are now available for some tumours, and treatments based on their use are under study. Studies with such products of the immune defence system as interferon and the interleukins (see Section 2) have not had the impact originally expected, but a more recent product, tumour necrosis factor (TNF), appears to have more value, especially when used in combination with other anti-cancer agents.

Genetic engineering

New techniques of molecular DNA biology offer a different approach in combating cancer. It may soon be possible to change the structure of DNA in cells and thus change the nature of actually or potentially malignant cells into cells without the properties of malignant growth. The new science of genetic engineering also has potential for changing the basic nature of cells to prevent cancer developing or to change the nature of malignant cells.

Combined genetic engineering and immunotherapy

Another approach using genetic engineering and immunology is already under study. In these studies genetic engineering techniques are used to change antibody-forming cells in mice to produce human cancer antibodies; these appear to be effective and safe to use against certain malignant cells. Trials of treatment of non-Hodgkin's lymphoma using this approach are currently under study, but many problems need to be addressed before such approaches are likely to be available for clinical use. One of these problems is the high cost of producing such antibodies.

Improved palliative care

For those people with advanced cancer and in great discomfort or pain, methods of relieving the suffering are now better understood. Such measures are now more readily available and there is little need for patients to suffer greatly from pain or other distressing symptoms of cancer. These facilities will be further improved and made more readily available to those who need them.

Hope for the future

For those with serious but not terminal disease, there are now good prospects for recovery: there is a probability of cure for increasing numbers of patients with cancer. Even for those with what is now considered to be terminal disease, worthwhile palliation is available to improve quality of life; and there remains the hope that for some, further improvement in treatment methods may soon bring a better prospect of cure.

Glossary

ACUTE
Having a sudden, severe and short course.

ADENOMA
A benign (not malignant) tumour in which the cells are derived from glands or from glandular epithelium such as the lining of the stomach.

ANAEMIA
A blood condition with reduced numbers of red blood cells and/or amount of haemoglobin.

Pernicious anaemia: A type of anaemia resulting from a failure of gastric mucosa (stomach lining) to produce a vital ingredient for making blood called 'intrinsic factor'.

ANOREXIA
A feeling of not wanting to eat (lack of hunger).

ANTIBODY
A particle manufactured in the immune system to defend the body against a harmful invading organism or particle called an antigen.

ARTERIOGRAM
A radiograph (X-ray photograph) of an artery taken after injection of a radio-opaque substance (dye) into the artery.

ASPIRATION
Act of sucking up or sucking out.

ASTROCYTOMA
A malignant tumour of connective tissue cells in the brain.

ATROPHIC
Wasted; degenerate; showing a loss of special qualities (adjective).

ATROPHY
Wasting away; losing special qualities (verb or noun).

AXILLA
Armpit.

BACTERIA
Germs.

BARIUM
A barium meal: A chalky, porridge-like substance containing the radio-opaque element, barium, which is swallowed to allow radiographs to be taken allowing the outline, size and shape of such organs as the stomach or duodenum to be seen on X-ray films or on an X-ray screen.

A barium swallow: Similar to a barium meal except that as the material is swallowed, X-ray films and screening of the oesophagus allows the shape and outline of the oesophagus to be studied.

A barium enema: Similar to a barium meal except the material is passed via a tube through the anus to allow X-ray films and screening of the rectum and large bowel.

BASAL	Basic. The lowest or foundation part of a structure. The basal layer of skin cells consists of the deeper cells from which the surface cells grow.
BCC	Basal cell carcinoma. A slowly growing skin cancer that grows from the deep (basal) layer of skin cells
BCG	Bacille Calmette-Guerin – a preparation originally used as an active immunising agent against tuberculosis. It consists of harmless living organisms that promote a similar body defence action to that of tuberculosis bacteria.
BENIGN	Not malignant; favourable for recovery; unlikely to be dangerous.
BENIGN MAMMARY DYSPLASIA	A condition of the breasts that is likely to cause cysts and other benign lumps in the breasts.
BIOPSY	The removal of a small sample of body tissue for microscopic examination.
BUCCAL MUCOSA	The lining of the cheek in the mouth.
CANCER	A malignant growth of cells; a continuous, purposeless, unwanted and uncontrolled growth of cells.
CAPSULE	The fibrous or membranous sac-like covering that encloses a tissue or organ.
CARCINOGEN	A substance that causes cancer.
CAT	See CT scan.
CERVIX UTERI	The neck of the uterus. The entrance of the womb.
CHEMOTHERAPY	Treatment with chemical agents or drugs.
CHRONIC	Persisting for a long time. Having a long or protracted course.

CHRONIC ATROPHIC GASTRITIS	A gradual and persistent degeneration of the lining of the stomach.
CONGENITAL	Present from the time of birth.
CORYNEBACTERIUM PARVUM	A harmless bacterium sometimes used to stimulate immune body defence reactions.
CROHN'S DISEASE	This name applies to granular colitis, an infection affecting the large bowel, or to a similar inflammatory condition which may affect the small intestine. The condition was first described by Dr Crohn.
CT SCAN (CAT SCAN OR COMPUTERISED AXIAL TOMOGRAPHY)	A method of visualising body tissues by using special computerised radiographic techniques to give X-ray 'pictures' of sections of body tissues.
CYTOTOXIC	Having a toxic or harmful effect upon cells.
DNA	Deoxyribonucleic acid – the material from which the body building genes and chromosomes are made.
ENDOSCOPE	An instrument used for visual examination of the interior of hollow organs or the interior of body cavities.
EPIDEMIOLOGY	The branch of medicine dealing with the distribution and incidence of disease and causes and spread of diseases.
EPIDEMIOLOGICAL	To do with epidemiology.
EPITHELIUM	Tissue that forms a body surface-lining such as skin surface or lining of a hollow organ that opens on to a body surface such as the lining of the mouth, bladder, bowel or vagina.
ESOPHAGUS	Same as oesophagus; the gullet.
FAECES	Bowel motion; stool.
FAMILIAL POLYPOSIS COLI	An inherited condition in which about half of the members of a family will develop polyps (small tumours) in the wall of the large bowel. Eventually one or more of these will become malignant.
FASCIA	Superficial fascia: the fatty layer under the skin.

Fascia or deep fascia: the fibrous or membranous layer of tissue that covers muscles, nerves and blood vessels, or separates muscles or other tissues into different compartments.

FIBROMA A benign tumour composed of fibrous tissues and fibrous tissue-forming cells.

FLOOR OF MOUTH The lower part of the mouth under the tongue.

GASTROSCOPE An instrument used for visual examination of the interior of the stomach.

GLAND A tissue or organ that manufactures and secretes chemical substances necessary for maintenance of normal health and body function.

GLUCAN A complex carbohydrate (type of sugar) that constitutes much of the fibre in common vegetable and grain foodstuffs and has been found to have immune stimulatory properties.

GOITRE Enlargement of the thyroid gland causing a swelling in the front part of the neck.

GRANULAR COLITIS (CROHN'S DISEASE) A type of chronic inflammatory condition of the large bowel of no known cause.
See Crohn's disease.

HRT (HORMONE REPLACEMENT THERAPY) Treatment with a low dose of hormones to reduce menopausal and postmenopausal symptoms and other problems such as loss of calcium from bones.

HYPERKERATOSIS A thickening of the flat protective surface layer of epithelium of skin or lip. The condition is usually characterised by a formation of a crust or flakes that drop off. There can be a tendency for malignant changes to appear gradually, and cancer may develop.

IMMUNOTHERAPY The treatment of disease by giving immune substances or by stimulating the immune system of body defences.

INDURATION The hardening or thickening of a tissue or a part of the body such as due to inflammation or infiltration with cancer.

LEUCOCYTE　　White cell. The 'white' or colourless type of cell that circulates in the blood, has amoeboid movement, and is chiefly concerned with defending the body against invasion of foreign organisms or bacteria.

LEUKOPLAKIA　　White patch. A disease distinguished by the presence of white thickened patches in the mucous membranes commonly in the mouth. There may be a tendency for malignant characteristics to appear gradually and thus for a cancer to develop.

LIPOMA　　A benign tumour composed of fat cells.

LIVER　　The largest solid organ in the body. It lies in the upper abdomen predominantly on the right side and under cover of the lower right ribs.

LYMPHANGIOGRAM　　A radiograph (X-ray photograph) of lymphatic vessels shown after injection of a radio-opaque substance (dye) into the lymphatic vessels.

LYMPHOCYTE　　One of the types of white cells that circulate in the blood and take part in immune reactions and the body's defence reactions. A mononuclear-non-granular leucocyte produced by lymph nodes and other lymphoid tissue.

LYMPHOID　　Resembling or pertaining to the tissue of the lymphatic system. Tissue that contains large numbers of round cells and produces lymphocytes.

LYMPHOMA　　A malignant tumour or cancer of lymphoid tissue.

LYMPH NODES　　Small masses of lymphatic tissue 1–15 mm in diameter and normally bean-shaped. Scattered along the course of lymph vessels and often grouped in clusters, they form an important part of the body's defence system, functioning as factories for the development of lymphocytes and filtering bacteria and foreign debris from tissue fluid. They are sometimes referred to as 'lymph glands'.

LYMPH VESSELS or LYMPHATICS　　The small vessels that drain tissue fluid into lymph nodes and inter-connect groups of lymph nodes. Eventually the larger lymph vessels drain this fluid into the bloodstream.

MALAISE　　A general feeling of lassitude and ill-health.

MALIGNANT	Life-threatening. A condition which in the natural course of events would become progressively worse, resulting in death. A malignant growth or cancer is a growth of unwanted cells that tends to continue growing and invade, thus destroying surrounding tissues. It also tends to spread to other parts of the body, destroying other tissues.
MALIGNANT FIBROUS HISTIOCYTOMA	A malignant tumour of histiocytes which are protective (immune) cells in soft tissues (muscles, fat etc.) or in bone.
MEDIASTINUM	The central midline area of the chest. That part of the chest between the sternum (breast bone) and the vertebrae (back bone). That part of the chest containing the heart, great blood vessels, trachea and oesophagus.
MEDULLOBLASTOMA	An uncommon malignant tumour that usually develops from primitive brain cells in the cerebellar part of the brain, most commonly in children and young people.
MELANOMA	A malignant growth (cancer) of pigment-producing cells most commonly arising in the skin, sometimes in the eye and occasionally elsewhere.
METASTATIC	Metastatic cancer is a secondary growth of malignant cells that has spread from a primary cancer elsewhere.
MONOCLONAL	An adjective that describes a particle of one special type only. A monoclonal antibody will affect one special chemical particle only, and therefore the special type of cell that carries this particle.
MRI	Magnetic resonance imaging. A special test based on certain laws of physics. The test allows X-ray like pictures to be taken of cross-sections of the body, head or limbs. The resulting pictures are rather like those of CT scans.
MUCUS	A protective slimy material secreted by certain glands and certain cells lining body cavities and hollow organs.

MUCOUS MEMBRANE   The lining of most hollow organs and some body cavities such as the mouth, stomach and bowel, all of which contain mucous glands and secrete mucus on to the surface.

NAEVUS (or NEVUS)   A localised collection of pigment-forming skin cells forming a localised and circumscribed malformation, usually pigmented, brown in colour, such as a mole or a birthmark.

NEOPLASM   Newgrowth. An abnormal growth of body cells. A neoplasm may be benign (usually harmless) with limited growth, or malignant, with continuous, unwanted, unlimited and uncontrolled growth (cancer).

NEPHROBLASTOMA   A type of kidney cancer that occurs in infants; sometimes called Wilm's tumour.

NEUROBLASTOMA   A malignant tumour of nerve-forming cells that usually arises in a special part of the nervous system called the autonomic nervous system.

NEUROMA   A benign tumour composed of nerve cells.

OESOPHAGUS (or Esophagus)   The part of the digestive tract for passage of food from the mouth and pharynx to the stomach below; a muscular tube lined with epithelium and extending from the neck through the chest and into the abdomen.

ONCOGENE   A particular gene in a person's chromosomes that can change and become responsible for tumour cell growth or cancer.

ONCOLOGY   The study of tumours, or the study of patients suffering from tumours.

OSTEOMYELITIS   Infection of bone.

PALLIATIVE   Giving relief. Relieving symptoms but not curing the condition.

PALLIATION   Relief.

PANCREAS   A pale fleshy gland that lies across the back of the abdominal cavity, mostly behind the stomach, responsible for secreting digestive substances into the digestive tract and insulin into the bloodstream (see Figure 1).

PAPILLOMA	A benign wart-like or fern-like tumour derived from epithelium and projecting from an epithelial lining of a surface with a central core of small blood vessels.
PET SCAN	Positron emission tomography. A special technique producing 'pictures' of body tissues based on different biochemical activity in the tissues.
PHYTOESTROGENS	Naturally occurring oestrogen-like hormones present in relatively large quantities in certain leguminous plants such as soy beans. Thought to be at least partly responsible for the lower incidence of some cancers (especially of the breast and the prostate) in people such as Asians who have a high intake of legumes in their diets.
PLATELETS	Small disc-shaped particles in the blood that are essential for blood clotting.
PLEURA	The lining or membrane surrounding the lungs and surrounding the cavity in which the lungs move during respiration.
POLYP	A tumour projecting on a stalk from the mucous membrane lining the cavity of a hollow organ.
PMS	Premenstrual symptoms of tension, mood changes, often depression, breast engorgement and pain and discomfort experienced a few days before menstruation.
PROSTHESIS	An artificial replacement for a missing part.
PROSTHETIC	To do with a prosthesis.
RADICAL	Extreme. A radical mastectomy is the surgical removal of the breast together with other nearby tissues.
RADIO-OPAQUE MATERIAL	A substance that does not allow penetration of X-rays, thus showing as a white area on an X-ray film. It is commonly referred to as 'dye'. Barium and iodine are radio-opaque substances often used in X-ray studies. Lead and other metals are also radio-opaque and prevent penetration by X-rays.
RADIOTHERAPY	Treatment with X-rays or gamma rays.

RETICULO-ENDOTHELIAL SYSTEM	Part of the immune system; the body system which consists of tissue defensive cells that protect the body against foreign materials and invading organisms. The special defensive cells are predominantly found in bone marrow, spleen, liver and lymph nodes but are also found in other tissues such as skin and soft tissues and the wall of stomach and bowel.
SARCOMA	A cancer of connective tissues such as muscle, fat, fascia or bone.
SCREENING TEST	A relatively simple, safe and easily performed test that can be carried out on large numbers of people to determine whether they are likely to have a cancer or other serious disease.
SIDE EFFECT	An effect other than the effect wanted.
SIGMOIDOSCOPE	A long, thin instrument used for passing through the anus with a light to allow visual examination of the inside of the lower bowel.
SPLEEN	A vascular solid organ in the upper left abdomen under the protection of the lower left ribs. Its main function is to filter old or damaged blood cells from the bloodstream (see Figure 1).
SQUAMOUS	Flat, like a scale or pavement. Squamous cells are flat scale-like cells that cover the skin, the mouth, throat, oesophagus, vagina and some other body cavities.
THERAPY	Treatment.
TISSUE	A layer or group of cells of particular specialised types that together perform a special function.
TOXIC	Poisonous.
TRAUMA	Injury.
TRAUMATISED	Injured.
TUMOUR (or TUMOR)	A swelling; the term commonly used to describe a swelling caused by a growth of cells – a newgrowth or neoplasm – that may be a cancer.
ULCERATIVE COLITIS	An inflammatory condition of the large bowel characterised by small ulcers in the bowel lining and causing episodes of diarrhoea.

UTERUS
The womb. The organ in the female pelvis in which a foetus develops.

VARICOSE ULCER
An ulcer in the skin, usually on the lower leg, caused by poor circulation in the tissues as a result of longstanding varicose veins.

Index

197

leukoplakia, 12, 26, 116, 117, 134, 176
lifestyle, 4, 21, 92, 176
limbs, 42, 50, 54, 59, 67, 77, 84
linear accelerator, 159
lining cells, 3, 7
lipoma, 13, 26, 162, 165
liposarcoma, 162, 164, 165, 167
lips, 11, 117, 118, 119, 124, 125
liquid nitrogen, 60, 67
liver, 3, 4, 8, 14, 19, 22, 32, 41, 47, 50, 53, 67, 70, 82, 91, 92, 94, 100, 103–106, 107, 108, 111, 112, 115, 127, 137, 144, 151, 156, 158, 159, 161, 173, 174, 180
liver scan, 92, 101, 114
local effects of cancer, 29
Lost Cords club, 123
lump, 30, 33, 89, 90, 113, 115, 116, 118, 119, 120, 121, 125, 126, 127, 134, 137, 142, 144, 145, 160, 166, 168, 171, 172
lungs, 3, 4, 5, 10, 16, 20, 22, 25, 29, 31, 32, 37, 38, 42, 53, 54, 60, 69, 70, 82, 84, 85, 86, 88, 91, 92, 104, 127, 135, 136, 144, 145, 151, 156, 163, 164, 167, 168, 173, 174
lymph nodes, 10, 30, 32, 34–35, 41, 42, 53, 54, 58, 78, 80, 81, 82, 83, 85, 91, 93, 94, 98, 100, 107, 114, 116, 117, 118, 119, 120, 121, 122, 123, 125, 126, 127, 129, 130, 134, 135, 136, 138, 143, 151, 155, 156, 157, 158–159, 160, 161, 163, 164, 166, 173, 174
lymph vessels, 2, 83, 162, 163, 173
lymphangiography, 41, 161
lymphangiosarcoma, 163
lymphatic leukaemia, 10, 35, 146
lymphocytes, 66, 149, 155
lymphoid tissue, 149, 156
lymphoma, 10, 31, 35, 40, 53, 63, 64, 110, 127, 156–162, 178
lymphoscintigrams, 159

M

macrophages, 66
magnetic fields, 44
malaise, 158
Malayia, 17
malaria, 19
Male, 13–141
male breast, 14, 63, 90, 136
malignant fibrous histiocytoma, 163, 165, 167

malnutrition, 32
mammary dysplasia, 12
mammography, 37, 39, 40, 91
marijuana, 176
masculising, 63
mass, 113
mastectomy, 57
mastectomy club, 96
mastitis, 12, 191
meat, 16–17, 22–23, 25, 100, 111
meditation, 70, 72, 74
medullary, 127
medulloblastoma, 10, 146, 148
melanoma, 11, 17, 18, 22, 25, 52, 64, 67, 73, 77, 81–84, 82, 87, 104, 133, 174, 177
men, 21, 63, 82, 84, 134–141
meninges, 146, 152
meningitis, 151, 152
menopause, 89, 90, 130, 133
menstruation, 89, 132
mental state, 69, 74
mesothelioma, 20, 87
metal workers, 20
metastatic, see secondary
methadone, 71
microscopic examination, 34, 36, 50, 51, 80, 82, 86, 97, 119, 126, 127, 130, 133, 137, 142, 158, 160, 166, 168, 169, 170, 171
microwaves, 67
milk, 17
moles, 26, 52, 82, 83
monoclonal antibodies, 181
morphine, 71, 75
mosquitoes, 19
mouth, 3, 5, 7, 11, 12, 21, 22, 25, 30, 31, 34, 35, 53, 55, 59, 68, 81, 96, 97, 110, 117, 118, 119, 123, 124, 174
MRI, 36, 43, 44, 147, 166, 168, 170, 171, 178
mucus, 121
mucus membrane, mucosa, 68, 81, 97, 117, 119
multiple myeloma, 63, 171
muscle, 3, 13, 30, 33, 67, 174
Muslims, 23
mustard gas, 56
myelogram, 38
myeloid leukaemia, 148, 149
myosarcoma, 163

pituitary gland, 62, 63
placenta, 131
plastic surgery, 54, 118
plastic tube, 98
platelets, 59, 153, 154, 155
pleura, 47, 69, 87
pleural cavity, 69, 88, 173
PMS, 23, 92
pneumonia, 4, 32, 69, 85, 151
pollutants, 177
polyp, 7, 8, 9, 12, 13, 26, 37, 47, 99,
    111, 176
postnasal space, 17, 45, 121
potassium, 49
pre-existing, 7, 116
pregnancy, 43, 60, 131, 150
pre-malignant conditions, 26, 47, 67, 128,
    134, 176
pre-menopausal, 23, 61
preservatives, 16, 99
pressure, 70, 146, 148
prevention, 25, 92, 133, 175
primary cancer, 30, 87, 88, 103–104, 105,
    127, 173
proctoscope, 46
progesterone, 63, 130
prostate, 3, 10, 15, 17, 23, 26, 32, 35, 48,
    50, 53, 60, 61, 69, 135, 136–141
prosthesis, 169
prostitutes, 24
PSA, 49, 138
psychiatrists, psychiatry, 25, 71–72
psychology, psychological factors, 16,
    24–25, 71–72
psychosomatic, 24
psychotherapy, 71
puberty, 11, 82
pubis, pubic bone, 129, 135
pump, 106, 115
punch out biopsy, 50, 138

Q

quacks, 5, 72, 74
quality of life, 115

R

race, 4, 7, 16, 17–18, 99, 149
radiation, 20, 150, 177
radiation field, 55, 57
radical mastectomy, 54, 93
radical operation, 116, 119, 120, 134, 140,
    172, 173

radio opaque material (dye) 39, 40, 41, 47
radioactive iodine, 41, 127
radioisotopes, 41–42, 126, 136, 147, 177
radiologist, 39
radiosensitive, 146
radiotherapist, 54, 93
radiotherapy, 53, 54–55, 57, 58, 59, 61, 69,
    70, 78, 80, 84, 86–87, 93–94, 95, 98, 110,
    115, 116, 118, 119, 120, 122–123, 124,
    125, 127, 129, 130, 133, 134, 136, 139,
    140, 141, 143, 145, 146, 148, 150, 151,
    152, 153, 155, 156, 159, 160, 161, 166,
    168, 169, 170, 171, 172, 179, 180
reconstructive surgery, 54, 96, 118
rectum, 9, 12, 14, 16, 26, 35, 38, 45, 54,
    100, 104, 105, 113, 114, 129, 132, 137,
    138, 143
recurrent cancer, 52, 73, 114, 123, 124,
    125, 163, 164, 166, 170
red blood cells, 48, 151
refrigeration, 16, 103
regional chemotherapy, 57, 59, 66, 81, 84,
    119, 141, 167, 169, 180
regression of cancers, 72, 74, 167
relaxation, 72
religion, 16–17, 23, 75
remission, 152
renal pelvis, 144, 145
repair, 5
research, 5
residual cancer, 73
rest, 69
retrograde pyelogram, 38
retrovirus, 5
rhabdomyosarcoma, 163, 164
Rocky Mountains, 20
rodent ulcer, 78
roughage, 16, 23
Russia, Russian, 97

S

sacrum, 129, 135
salivary glands, 3, 123–125
sarcomas, 13, 54, 59, 88, 127,
    162–173, 174
scan, 126, 127, 136, 138, 145, 147, 159, 161
Scandinavia, 17, 97, 149
SCC, 18, 52, 77, 79–81, 82, 116, 117,
    128, 134
sciatica, sciatic nerve, 137
scientific analysis, 74

scintigraphy, 83
screening test, screening clinic, 34, 36, 53, 91, 128, 177
scrotum, 6, 34, 135
second cancer, 7, 112
secondaries, 2, 4, 30, 40, 52, 67, 70, 85, 87–88, 91, 95, 104– 105, 111, 114, 115, 120, 127, 133, 135, 136, 137, 138, 139, 140, 145, 158, 167, 168, 173–174
selenium, 26
self-examination, 30, 37
serum tests, 36, 48, 177
Seventh Day Adventists, 16–17
sex, sexual activity, 4, 61, 62
sexual organs, cancer of, 128–141
siblings, 150, 153
side effects, 56, 59, 62, 63, 68, 139, 140, 160, 178
sigmoidoscope, 45, 113
signs, 33
sinus, 117
size of tumour, 30
skin, 3, 6, 7, 8, 11, 14, 17, 18, 20, 25, 30, 31, 34, 52–53, 55, 59, 67, 69, 77–84, 87, 95, 111, 116, 117, 134, 156, 160, 173, 174, 177
skin lotions, 25
skull, 121, 122
small bowel, 47, 101–102, 110, 111
smell, 147
smoked fish, 16, 99
smoking, 5, 7, 10, 12, 16, 17, 21, 22, 25, 84–85, 89, 99, 107, 117, 120, 122, 141, 176
social habits, 16, 23
social workers, 24, 72
soft tissue tumours, 26, 30, 88, 162–167
soot, 6
South Africa, 17, 18, 97
soy, 15, 23, 90, 137, 176
speaking difficulty, 31
speech, 147
sperm, spermatozoa, 60
spices, 99
spinal cord, 38, 70
spiritual help, 71, 72
spleen, 35, 41, 108, 149, 151, 154, 156, 158, 159, 160, 174
spread, 30, 44, 53, 58, 82, 109, 124, 127, 129, 131, 135, 139, 173

sputum, 31, 85, 86
staging laparotomy, 157
starch, 16
sterility, 60
stomach, 3, 5, 8, 9, 10, 11, 13, 14, 16, 21, 22, 25, 31, 32, 34, 37, 38, 45, 47, 53, 54, 59, 69, 97, 98, 99–103, 104, 105, 108, 109, 123, 133, 156, 160, 163, 164, 174, 176, 177
stones, 12, 26, 144
stress, 16, 24
sublingual, 124
submandibular, 124
suicide, 76
sunburn, 11, 18, 25
sunlight hypersensitivity, 68
sunshine, 6, 11, 14, 17, 18, 19, 22, 25, 77–78, 79, 82, 118, 176
surgery, 53, 59, 61, 78, 80, 86, 92, 93–94, 95, 98, 101–102, 104, 106, 116, 119, 120, 122, 124, 125, 126, 127, 129, 130, 134, 135, 140, 141, 143, 145, 148, 158, 166, 167, 169, 170, 171, 172, 180
swallowing difficulty, 31, 32, 97
swelling, 30, 33, 70, 113, 132, 135–136, 168, 170, 171
switching off mechanism, 1, 5
Switzerland, 20
symptoms, 29, 33
synovial sarcoma, 163, 165

T

tamoxifen, 61–62, 92, 94
target tumour cells, 179
tars, 6, 10
taxanes, 178
tear duct, 79
teenagers, 10, 82, 89, 126
television X-ray screening, 39
tendons, 162
testis, 10, 13–14, 34, 134–136
thorascopy, 47
throat, 3, 5, 11, 12, 21, 22, 25, 30, 31, 34, 35, 45, 55, 59, 117, 118, 120, 121, 123, 174
thrombosis, 63, 151
thyroglossal cyst, 13
thyroid, 3, 17, 19, 41, 50, 63, 125–127
thyroxine, 63, 125, 126, 127
tired, 100, 112, 142, 147, 154
TNF, 64, 66, 84, 181